The Bodyweight Exercise Bible: Bodyweight Workout Routines For Men And Women

By Anthony Anholt

Copyright © 2013 By Anthony Anholt

Discover other fitness titles by Anthony Anholt on Amazon:

The Isometric Exercise Bible

Disclaimer

The exercises and advice contained within this course may be too strenuous or dangerous for some people and the reader(s) should consult a physician before engaging in them. The author and publisher of this book are not responsible in any manner whatsoever for any injury which may occur through reading and following the instructions herein.

Table Of Contents

How Changing Your Body Can Change Your Life

You are never given a wish without being given the power to make it true. You may have to work for it, however -Richard Bach

I have a question for you. Are you happy with your life right now? If I gave you a magic wand which facets of your life would you improve today? There are many qualities that form a well-lived and fulfilling life. Family, occupation, hobbies and friends are just a few of the things you might think of if I asked you to make a list. Although most people often mentally separate these elements into their own separate boxes the reality is that they are all interconnected. Money pressures, for example, can put strains on a marriage whereas family strife can bleed into work and other areas. But if I asked you to pick one aspect that forms a foundation of a happy, the one from which everything else flows, which would you choose? In my opinion there is only one choice and that is your health.

Think about it. How can you enjoy your family if you are sick? How productive can you be at work if you feel tired all the time? How confident can you be if you are physically weak? I can't think of a single characteristic of a happy life that is not built upon a foundation of being healthy enough to enjoy it; it is the foundation on which everything else rests. When you have your health the world opens up to you and life is full of possibilities. Without it the world is a much smaller and darker place.

Now let's take this idea and go a step further. Imagine right now that you are not only healthy but you possess it to a superior degree. You are strong, fit and possess a boundless, youthful energy along with an extreme mental clarity. Compared to your peers you stand out in an almost superhuman way. If you are older people routinely mistake you for being 10 to 20 years younger than you really are. If you are younger people simply marvel at your strength, athletic ability and vitality. People from all walks of life are almost magnetically drawn to the energy you effortlessly radiate. Can you not see how this would positively affect and improve every other aspect of your life? Closed doors would open and you'd have the strength and confidence to walk through them. You would interact with other people with deserved confidence and pride. Life would simply becoming easier as well as more exciting as it opened up with possibilities. Transforming your body can literally transform your life. It really is that simple.

How Bodyweight Exercises Can Transform Your Body

The only person stopping you from having the body and life you want to have is the person you see when you look in the mirror.

Now take a moment and imagine your dream body - what does it look like? If you're like most people you probably find the freakish, steroid enhanced muscles of the professional bodybuilder to be utterly unappealing. More likely you are drawn to the natural physiques that professional dancers, gymnasts and martial artists possess. What is the common thread that binds these kinds of physiques together? The answer is that to one extent or another they all train naturally using nothing but their own body and bodyweight. They don't use weights or fancy equipment of any kind. Why does this method of exercise yield such desirable results?

One reason is that our muscles are designed to work together as a unit. By their nature this is exactly how bodyweight workouts train the body. This not only creates an extremely powerful and functional physique but one that is symmetrical and pleasing to look at as well. This gives you a natural, healthy look that screams good health.

As an example of this concept consider what is probably the most famous and effective bodyweight exercise of them all, namely the classic pushup. When you perform a pushup you are primarily working your chest, back and arm muscles. Now, let's say that your arms are relatively weaker compared to your chest and back. Which muscle group will get the most work and tire first when you perform a pushup? You guessed it, your arms. Moreover, as you continue to do pushups your arms will gain strength faster relative to your chest and back until they reach parity. Not only is this visually pleasing but it is highly functional as well. This is why people who engage in bodyweight training are much less susceptible to injury as opposed to those who do not.

Another reason that bodyweight training has the ability to quickly transform your physique is that it is the best at building and maintaining your fast twitch muscle fibers. These are the fibers that keep you strong, athletic and youthful. Here's why.

Essentially your muscles are made up of two kinds of muscle fibers, fast twitch and slow twitch. The fast twitch fibers are larger and more powerful than their slow twitch counterparts but they tire out much more quickly. These are the muscles that you use when engaging in intense activities like jumping or lifting heavy objects. They are primarily fueled by glycogen (sugar) that is stored in the muscle itself. Slow twitch muscle fibers are smaller and weaker but possess much greater endurance. Think of a chicken. The legs, which are used for the endurance activity of walking, contain the dark meat. The breasts, on the other hand, are used for the intense activity of flapping the wings. The meat here is white and sweet due to the glycogen that is stored in them.

Simply put the more fast twitch muscle fibers you possess the younger and more dynamic you will be. Compare the physiques of sprinters to long distance marathon runners. The sprinters are invariably ripped and look younger than they really are. They move with the grace of panthers. Marathon runners, on the other hand, invariably look older and weaker. The reason for this is that the short and intense activity of sprinting builds fast twitch muscle fibers whereas marathon runners only make use of slow twitch fibers. As their training doesn't make use of them marathon runners literally lose their fast twitch muscle fibers overtime. By engaging in short bursts of intense bodyweight training you will be building fast twitch muscle fibers. This is the key to staying young and powerful.

Real Bodyweight Strength Vs. Phony Gym Strength

Be who you were created to be, and you will set the world on fire - St. Catherine of Sienna

Another big advantage that bodyweight training has over traditional gym workouts is that you gain real, functional strength. What is functional strength? It simply means the strength to perform any task you ask of your body with ease and grace. This could be simply carrying the groceries or playing a great game of tennis. You live your life using your body, not lifting weights. Weight lifting prepares you to lift more weights; bodyweight exercises prepare you for life.

Again, think of gymnasts. They don't train with weights at all yet they can go into a gym and throw weight around like nobodies business. What is more damming is that the opposite is not true. A gymnast can do what a weight lifter can do, but a weight lifter will be dead hopeless at performing a simple gymnastic posture. Karl Gotch, a famous old time professional wrestler (when professional wrestling was real) is known to have called gym physiques counterfeit muscle. They may look like a million bucks but none of it is worth a damn. To excel in the real world you need the real thing, not a glossy imitation. This is what bodyweight exercises will give you.

Why Cardio Does NOT Help With Fat Loss

Health and good estate of body are above all gold, and a strong body above infinite wealth.
-Ecclesiasticus 30:15

One thing that will likely surprise you is how superior bodyweight workouts can be to traditional forms of cardio like jogging or riding an exercise bike when it comes to burning fat. This goes against the conventional wisdom that long slow cardio sessions are the key as they allow the body to burn fat directly. This is the reason you see so many people hunched over exercise bikes and stair masters in various gyms around the world. However, as with so many other things the conventional wisdom is wrong in this instance. Here's why.

When you are weighing the merits of various fat burning exercises you have to look at the big picture. You have to consider not only what happens when the exercise is being performed but also what happens afterwards when it is finished. It is true that low intensity exercise allows you to burn a greater percentage of fat while the exercise is being performed. The problem though is that as soon as you stop exercising so does the fat burning. When you engage in higher intensity short term exercise, the kind that works those fast twitch muscle fibers I was talking about, you burn more sugar and carbs as opposed to fat. When you stop exercising though your body will react by burning fat stores into order to replace the glycogen that was used up in your muscles.

This results in a metabolism boost that may last up to 48 hours after you finish your workout.

This phenomenon has actually been proven scientifically. Dr. Angelo Tremblay of the Physical Activities Science Laboratory in Quebec conducted a study comparing the benefits of low intensity, long duration exercise vs. high intensity, short duration. The results were clear. Not only did the high intensity/short duration group lose more body fat overall they lost it much more efficiently. Not only did they burn more fat when the workout was over but Dr. Tremblay found that high intensity/short duration workouts also suppressed the appetite.

The last reason that bodyweight workouts are so effective at burning fat is that they work multiple muscle groups at once. To demonstrate this consider that classic of gym-based workouts, the bench press. When you perform a bench press you are working your chest and arms muscles (and inefficiently at that). For the rest of your body though there is no difference between performing a bench press and lying in bed. Now contrast this to a pushup hitting those areas plus every other muscle group in your body to one extent or another, including your legs. This is why when it comes to burning fat bodyweight exercises really can't be beat.

Goal Setting, Your Mind And Getting The Results You Want

It's repetition of affirmations that leads to belief and once that belief becomes a deep conviction, things begin to happen. - Muhammad Ali

On your journey to the new you this section may be the most important, even more important than the exercises themselves. Although it is short it is absolutely critical and I don't think I'm exaggerating when I say your success or failure likely hinges on how well you absorb what I am about to reveal to you. Please read it carefully.

Now, I'm about to nerd out on you for a moment but stick with me. Imagine the starship Enterprise from Star Trek fame. If the Enterprise has a mission to reach a certain star system what are the most important items it needs to accomplish its goal? Well, it obviously needs enough fuel and the ship needs to be in good working order, but this is not the critical factor as by default Scotty is pretty good at maintaining the ship. No, the critical factor the ship needs is a destination to feed into the ships navigation computers. The navigation computers on the Enterprise are extremely powerful. Properly programmed they are guaranteed to get the Enterprise to its destination. If Kirk gets distracted (likely by some green alien woman) and forgets to set a course who knows where the Enterprise will wind up. It's a big universe.

Now here's the thing. When it comes to setting a course, you are not unlike the good ship Enterprise. You may not realize it at the moment, but you are actually in possession of a goal-setting computer that is even more powerful than the one that exists on the fictional Enterprise. Furthermore, your goal-setting computer is waiting to be tapped and is eager and willing to help you reach any goal you might have. As this book is concerned with bodyweight fitness and transforming your body, we are going to use it as a tool to help you reach the destination of your dream body.

What I am going to do now, in as little space as possible is explain how your goal-setting computer, your mind, actually works. I will then outline how to use it to get the results you want. What I am about to discuss falls under the "Law Of Attraction" as popularized by such books as, *The Secret* and *Think and Grow Rich*. If you want to learn more about what I am about to discuss, I have included a list of these works in the back of this book. For my money, the best and shortest book I've come across is, *It WORKS*, by RJH. Most of the following discussion is largely rooted in this work. I highly recommend it.

Let's go back to our Star Trek analogy, as your mind is not unlike the Enterprise. Your mind possesses a captain not unlike the famous and volatile Captain Kirk. You know it as your objective or conscious mind. This is the part of your mind that you are aware of right now. Ideas flow freely through it, often jumping from one concept to another within seconds. It is your conscious mind that makes decisions.

12

Do you exercise, get a drink of water, watch TV? This is your conscious mind, your captain, in action.

There is a second part of your mind that you may not be aware of although it exists just the same. Known as your subjective or unconscious mind it is roughly comparable to Scotty toiling away in the engine room. Although Kirk is the captain and gives the orders it is Scotty who actually operates the controls and carries them out. What is interesting though is that Scotty, working in the bowels of the ship, is essentially blind. He is completely dependent on the information and orders that Kirk relays to him. If Kirk gives an order to turn the ship hard to port to avoid an asteroid, for example, Scotty will carry out the order regardless if the asteroid actually exists or not. He is utterly dependent on the information that Kirk gives him.

As it is for Kirk and Scotty, so it is for your conscious and unconscious mind. Your conscious mind gives the orders and your unconscious mind blindly accepts them and attempts to carry them out, even when they may not be true. You can actually demonstrate this phenomenon by having an individual hold a weight in front of them for time. If you whisper in their ear beforehand "You are weak and useless, you are weak and useless" repeatedly they will hold the weight for considerably less time than if you say "You are strong and powerful, you are strong and powerful". This phenomenon has been proven scientifically over and over again. What is going on here? When the subconscious mind receives instructions from the conscious it acts on them, period. This is why it is so important to control what your objective mind is saying.

Here's what happens for most people, however. As they are not aware of the relationship between their conscious and unconscious minds they never make the effort to control what their objective mind is thinking. This results in the subjective mind receiving a steady stream of often completely contradictory orders. It's as if Captain Kirk is giving orders in rapid-fire fashion such as:

"Warp Factor 8"

"Raise The Shields"

"Full reverse on the engines"

"Transfer auxiliary power to the shields"

"Who's that green alien woman?"

"Red alert!"

"Clear the bridge!"

When faced with this steady stream of nonsense what would Scotty do? Most likely he would simply stop working until the orders became clearer. This is exactly what your subconscious mind does as well. When given contradictory or nonsense orders it simply ceases to function. This is what the legendary Muhammad Ali is referring to in the quote that started this chapter. *Thoughts lead to belief, which become deep convictions. When that occurs things begin to happen.*

Are you ready to make things happen?

Are you ready to get in the best shape of your life and reach your goals?

If so this is why we are going to spend a little bit of time mapping out a plan for to follow even before we get to the exercises. You will then use this plan, which from now on we will refer to as your dream body blueprint, to program your subconscious mind to reach your health and fitness goals.

Hold a picture of yourself long and steadily enough in your mind's eye, and you will be drawn toward it ~ Napoleon Hill

The first thing I want you to do is to find a picture of what represents your dream body to you. It could be an older picture of yourself when you were at your ideal weight. It could also be of a fitness model or celebrity whose physique you admire. It doesn't really matter where you get the picture from so long as the picture inspires you in some way. The picture you choose should make you think, "I want to look like this, this is who I want to be, this is why I exercise".

The reason the first thing I want you to do when constructing your blueprint is to find an inspiring image is that images are extremely powerful and useful when setting a course for your subconscious mind to follow. This is what the great Napoleon Hill is getting at in the quote above and why the saying, "A picture is worth a thousand words" is so true. When you start following this bodyweight fitness program there are going to be times when you just don't feel like doing it. This is natural and to be expected. We all have times when we feel lazy. The key though is to not let this feeling win. When you feel a wave of procrastination creeping over you think of this picture. Think of where you want to go and want you want to accomplish. What you will find is that simply thinking of this visual representation of your goal will be enough to get you back on track.

Next, get a piece of paper or fire up the word processor and paste this picture right at the top. Below it I want you to write down some goals related to what you need to do in order to start approaching your goal. To start off with I suggest you focus on process goals that you have complete control over as opposed to outcome goals for which you do not. For example, a process goal would be "I am going to get up early everyday so that I can exercise before work". This is doable and is completely under your control. A result goal would be "I am going to lose 5 pounds by April 11". These kinds of goals do have value and after a few months you can start setting goals such as this. The reason I do not recommend you start with them is that losing weight can be such an individual thing. You can be making great progress in getting healthy but the weight may not come off as you plan. You may then get discouraged and give up on the whole program, which would be a tragic mistake.

Are process goals, like loosing 5 pounds, not useful then? They are and here's how you use them. Once you have gotten used to hitting your individual process goals after a month or two you can start setting result goals. Always list your process goals first and your result goals with dates afterward. Here's how you should approach this. Your goal setting computer is like a guided missile. Your result goals are your target whereas your process goals are the means by which you achieve them (the fuel in the rocket engine, if you want to extend my analogy). So, you have your goal set and you launch the cruise missile. Did you hit your target? If so, congratulations! Time to set a new goal. What happens if you miss it? No worries there either. Just go back to your process goals and make the necessary adjustments. Perhaps you just need more time to reach your goal, or perhaps you need to adjust your workout routine. The key thing is now that you know what to do you shouldn't panic if you miss your target initially. In fact, don't view it negatively at all. See it as getting positive information back about what you need to do to reach your final destination.

When you are finished your personal Dream Body Blueprint should look something like this:

My Dream Body Blueprint

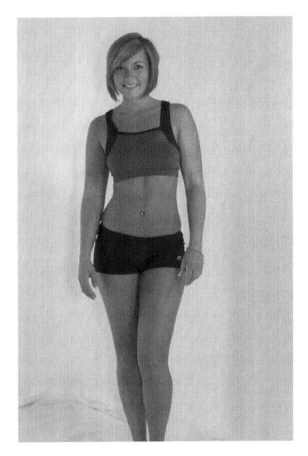

My Goals

- I am going to get up early at least five times a week and perform "The Fantastic Four" before work.
- I am going to start eating less sugary, processed food and more fruits and vegetables.
- I am going to read my dream body blueprint at least 3 times a day. When I am tired or don't feel like starting or finishing a workout I will picture my dream body image in my mind to motivate myself.

This is only an example but you get the idea. I realize you have no idea of what "The Fantastic Four" is yet but we will get to it. This list should be tailored to your own unique circumstances. You will want to carry this plan with you at all times. I say that you should read it three times a day (and I do recommend you make it a goal in your blueprint) but this is the bare minimum. If you have a few minutes while you're waiting in a line, for example, pull out your blueprint and read it. The more repeated and consistent the orders are that your subconscious mind receives overtime the better and quicker your results will be. You want to use this blueprint to set a course and stick to it!

One really cool thing you are likely to experience is that after following your blueprint for a while is that ideas will start to manifest themselves in your brain. Why is this? Essentially, this is your subconscious mind speaking to you. Your subconscious mind has access to the entire wealth of knowledge of the universe. When it accepts a clear goal it will use this knowledge to make suggestions to you. When these suggestions come you should heed them. Going back to our Star Trek analogy it's almost like Scotty calling the bridge and saying, "If we want to get to Vulcan, why don't we use the warp drive?"

Now that you have set a course by creating the all-important blueprint it is time to get to the actual exercise program. Are you ready to engage warp speed towards your goals? Then full speed Mr. Scott, maximum warp!

How To Use This Bodyweight Workout Program

Regardless of who you are or what you have been, you can be what you want to be - W. Clement Stone

The foundation of the Bodyweight Exercise Bible is something I like to call "The Fantastic Four". The Fantastic Four is made up of four pillars of exercise that, when taken together, form a firm foundation from which you will build the new, healthy you. Let's now look at each pillar in order to better understand why they are so important and why you should do them.

Pillar #1 – The Upper Body

The first pillar of the fantastic four is an exercise that will work your upper body. For this we turn to some variation of one of the most famous bodyweight exercises there is, namely the pushup. Pushups are a classic exercise that people have been doing since the times of ancient Greece if not before. The reason this exercise has lasted so long in its various forms is that it simply works. The classic pushup works your entire body (including your legs) but with a focus on your upper body including your chest, back and arms. Pushups force your entire body to work as a unit, which is exactly what we want. Some additional benefits of performing pushups include the following:

- The three ways in which you can work a muscle are with concentric motions, eccentric motions and isometric. Concentric muscle building occurs when the muscles are stimulated to contract. Eccentric muscle building occurs when a muscle becomes elongated due to a muscle opposite it contracting. Isometric muscle building occurs when a muscle attempts to contract but no movement occurs. When done properly pushups build muscle using all three methods.
- Like almost all bodyweight exercises pushups help train your proprioceptive muscle fibers that help to keep your body balanced. Pushups force these fibers to constantly work in order to prevent your body from tipping over. Training them will help you improve and maintain your sense of balance and speed overtime.
- Pushups help to train your body to recover faster after engaging in strenuous physical activity by encouraging blood flow. The soreness that is commonly associated with muscles after physical exertion is caused by the buildup of lactic acid. The increased blood flow that bodyweight workouts encourage helps to clear out the muscles thereby minimizing this effect.

Pillar #2 – The Lower Body

If we have an exercise for the upper body is only makes sense to follow it up with an exercise for the lower. In order to do this we turn to some form of the bodyweight squat. Bodyweight squats will provide you with all of the benefits that pushups do along with the following:

- Your legs contain the largest muscles in your body which makes them the most effective at burning fat by far. Do you want to burn fat? Work your legs!
- Powerful leg muscles will help you maintain a youthful spring in your step. When a professional athlete starts to age what is the first thing that typically goes on them? Their legs. It doesn't matter whether it's a boxer, basketball player or runner. By keeping your legs fresh bodyweight squats will help keep you young.
- Strong legs will help improve your circulation, which will help your heart. Blood circulation problems typically originate in the legs. Strong healthy legs make it easier for your heart to pump blood. There is a saying I've heard that says your legs can act like a second heart for your lower body. Strong legs and a healthy heart go hand-in-hand.
- Bodyweight squats will get you huffing and puffing which builds endurance and lungpower.

Pillar #3 – The Core

To most people few things scream fitness and health more than a tightly toned midsection. Beyond mere appearance however possessing a strong core is vital in building a truly functional body that can be worked in all directions and from all angles. A strong core is also vital in eliminating lower back pain and weakness, which so many people suffer from.

Pillar #4 – Back Bending

These kinds of exercises also work the core but more importantly they really strengthen your spine. There is an old saying in yoga that states *a healthy spine equals a healthy life* and this is very true. There is no more important body part to keep strong and healthy than your spine. Think about it. You can hurt your arm or pull a muscle and leg and still function. When you throw out your back however you immediately are transformed into an old man or woman in extremely poor health. Tasks as simple as standing up or walking become a struggle. Most people have poor backs because their core is weak to begin with. The less obvious reason is that so many of us spend so much time hunched over desks, which means we are constantly bending forward. This bent forward position causes tension to build up in the spine that can only be released through bending the back backwards. This is why there is so much emphasis put on back bending exercises in disciplines such as yoga. The spine is meant to be moved in all directions and it needs to bend backward to remain healthy.

How To Begin

When it comes to eating right and exercising there is no "'I'll start tomorrow." Tomorrow is a disease – V.L. Allinea

With the preliminaries out of the way you are probably eager to start your journey to becoming a better, healthier and stronger you. To begin with I suggest you start performing the fantastic four at a level appropriate for your fitness level for a least a month. This will ensure that your body is strong enough to start adding exercises later on. However if you feel you have mastered the beginner level feel free to move onto the intermediate or advanced levels whenever you see fit. You can exercise everyday if you feel up to it but so long as you workout three or four times a week you will make rapid progress.

One thing you will notice is that I never mention sets, meaning repeating the same exercise two or three times. You can perform these exercises in sets if you wish but I have found it to not really be necessary. Also I get bored easily and I would rather do a completely different exercise once than the same exercise over and over. Keeping my workouts fun and interesting is important to me, which is why I like variety. However, this is up to you.

One very important point that you need to remember is to never hold your breath when performing these exercises. You should always be striving to either breathe in through your nose or out through your mouth at all times. The reason for this is that holding your breath during intense physical activity causes your blood pressure to spike in unhealthy ways. This occurs because when your muscles are working hard they need oxygen. If you are not breathing though your heart attempts to compensate by pumping harder so that it can recycle the blood and oxygen it currently has in order to feed those muscles. This is not something you want to happen so make sure you are always breathing. Don't hold your breath!

When you breathe I generally recommend that you breathe in through your nose during the downward motion and out through your mouth when you reverse it. This is not written in stone, however. I know of many people who find it more comfortable to do the exact opposite. So, although I usually stress when I think you should breathe for the various exercises feel free to change it if something else works better for you. So long as you are not holding your breath you'll be fine.

One of the things that I love about bodyweight fitness exercises is that it is so easy to change and modify them. For example, let's take the classic pushup. How can this exercise be modified? Let's count the ways:

- Increase or decrease the leverage – By this I mean changing the angle at which the exercise is performed. If you perform a pushup with your feet raised on a platform, for example, it will become much harder.

- Use an unstable platform – If you have to constantly focus on your balance when you perform an exercise your muscles will have to work extra hard. Performing pushups on a pair of basketballs will accomplish this.
- Use isometric pauses – Simply pausing at the top or bottom of a movement and holding it for 5 to 7 seconds works your muscles in an isometric fashion.
- Vary the speed – Performing a pushup rapidly works your muscles differently than performing a very slow and controlled movement.
- Single limb movements – Where possible try performing the exercise using only a single limb. In the case of pushups this would mean performing a one-arm pushup.

As you can see you should never be bored with bodyweight exercises. The only thing limiting you is your imagination.

When you feel like quitting early or not even starting think of your dream body picture. This simple act of focusing on your goal should align your conscious and unconscious minds and get you in the mood to at least start your workout. The hardest part of any endeavor is often simply starting. Remember Zig Ziglar's advice:

When you don't really want to or feel like doing what needs to be done, do it and then you will feel like doing it. - Zig Ziglar

Once you have reached the advanced level of the fantastic four what comes next is really up to you. You can simply continue to workout with these exercises and you'll be in fantastic shape. However, if you want to take it to the next level or are simply looking for some variety I have included supplemental exercises for each of the four pillars. You can either add these exercises to the fantastic four as I've outlined or replace them entirely. It's up to you and the goals you've set for yourself. The key thing though is to have fun with it. You don't need to kill yourself with every workout. Remember, getting fit, much like life, is a marathon, not a sprint. Slow and steady wins the race. Ready to begin? Here's a quote from Dr. Seuss to get you on your way:

Today is your day, your mountain is waiting, so get on your way! – Dr. Seuss

The Fantastic Four – Beginner Level

Each person's task in life is to become an
increasingly
better person - Leo Tolstoy

If you are a complete beginner this is your starting point. Remember to take it slow and do what you can. If you haven't exercised in a long time you will likely be surprised at how challenging these bodyweight workouts are. However, if you stick to it, you will also likely be equally surprised at how fast your progress will be.

Pillar #1 (Beginner) – Upper Body - Beginner Pushup

The beginner pushup is an excellent upper body exercise to start with if you are not able to perform a regular pushup. When you can perform 25 beginner pushups in a row you should consider moving to a full pushup.

1. Begin on your knees with your hands out in front of you.
2. Take a deep breath through your nose as you lower yourself to the ground.
3. Exhale through you mouth as you press yourself back up to the starting position.

If you are not strong enough to lower yourself all the way to the ground simply go as far as you can. With time work on getting your chest low enough so that it touches the ground.

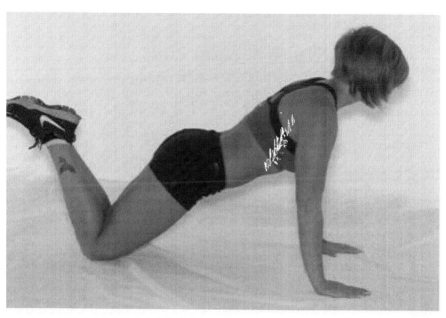

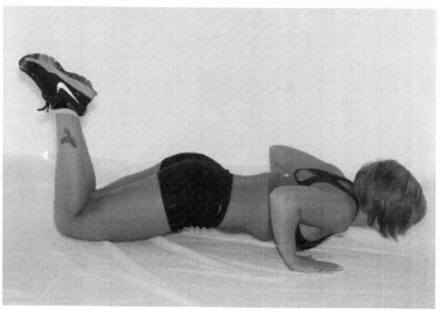

Pillar #2 (Beginner) – Lower Body – Bootstrappers

Bootstrappers are a squat variation that is ideal for beginners as your hands provide stability while reducing the amount of bodyweight you have to squat. Make sure you protect your lower back at all times by keeping your stomach sucked in and tight. If you feel any strain at all it is acceptable to keep your knees slightly bent in the "Up" position. When you can perform 50 bootstrappers in a row consider moving onto a more advanced exercise.

1. Begin by squatting down on the floor with your hands in front of you. Your knees should be together with your heels off the floor. Ideally, 60% of your weight should be on your legs with the rest on your hands.
2. Inhale through your nose as you straighten your legs until your heels touch the ground.
3. Exhale through your mouth as you bend your legs and return to the starting position.

As always, modify this movement so that you are comfortable. For example, if you are not flexible enough to straighten your legs so that your heels touch the ground simply go as far as you can.

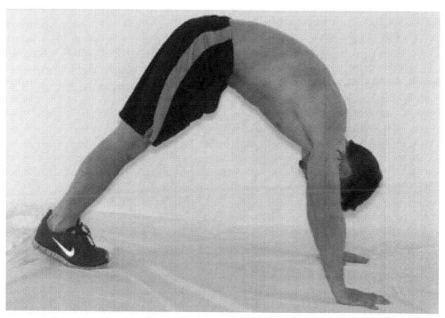

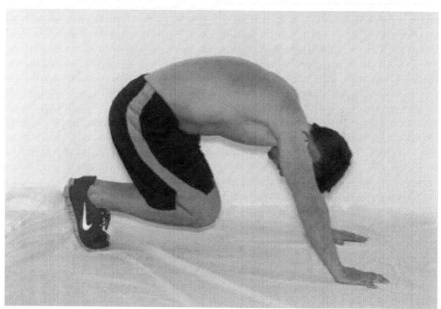

Pillar #3 (Beginner) – Core – The Rower

The rower is a fantastic exercise for building strong and lean abs. It will develop your entire abdominal region while simultaneously helping to eliminate any pain or weakness in your lower back. When you can perform 20 in a row you can consider moving up to the intermediate core exercise.

1. Lie down on your back with your arms by your sides.
2. Tuck your chin into your chest and tighten your stomach muscles.
3. Raise your upper body and legs simultaneously and bring them together. The closer you get your torso to your legs the more your abs are working.
4. Reverse the movement and return to the starting position.

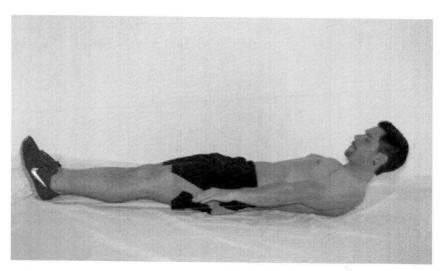

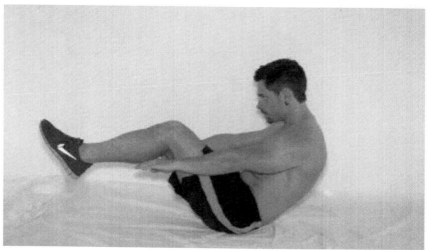

Pillar #4 (Beginner) – Back Bending – Ying/Yang Bends

For many of you this may be your first introduction to a back bending exercise. The key is to move slowly and deliberately while keepings your abs tight at all times, particularly for the forward bends. Keep your knees slightly bent at all times as this takes pressure off your lower back.

1. With your feet shoulder width apart and your knees slightly bent place your hands on your lower back.
2. Breathe in through your nose as you bend your back backwards, almost as if you are trying to look at the ceiling. Go as far as you can while maintaining your balance.
3. Exhale through your mouth as you bend forward at your waist trying to touch your hands to the floor. If you can't reach the floor or if you back is tight feel free to increase the bend in your knees.
4. Repeat this motion 10 times.

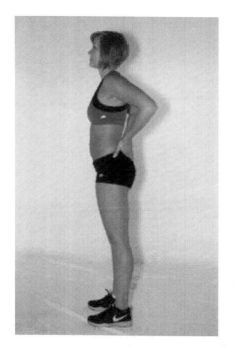
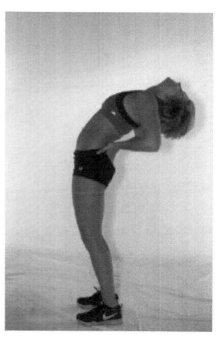
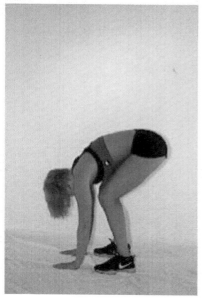

The Fantastic Four – Intermediate Level

If you have the courage to begin you have the courage to succeed – David Viscott

If you feel you have mastered the beginner level it's time to move onto the intermediate. You should already be feeling the enormous benefits that bodyweight workouts offer. Keep it up!

Pillar #1 (Intermediate) – Upper Body - Classic Pushup

There is a reason the pushup has been around for so long and is a favorite of athletes such as martial artists and gymnasts – it simply works. Pushups will help you build tremendous upper body strength while chiseling your shoulders, chest, and arms. When you perform this exercise keep your abs and glutes tight at all times. If your wrists bother you at all feel free to change your hand position to eliminate this feeling. Alternatively you can try putting your hands into a "fist" position with your knuckles on the ground. Doing so will completely eliminate the bend in your wrists but your may want to place a towel under your knuckles for comfort.

1. Lie face down on the ground with your legs straight behind you.
2. Stretch your arms straight out from your sides so that they are at a 90 degree angle from you body. Now bend your elbows to a 90-degree angle and rotate your shoulders until your palms are underneath your elbows. This is known as the 90/90 beginning pushup position.
3. Take a deep breath through your nose.
4. Press yourself off the floor as you exhale through your mouth.
5. Inhale as you lower yourself to the ground. Ideally you want your chest to touch the ground.

Always strive to keep your body as straight as a board when performing a pushup. Don't sag at the waist or stick your butt in the air. Do as many pushups as you can until fatigued.

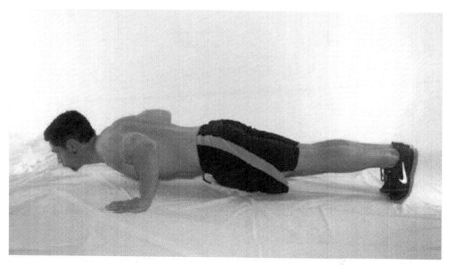

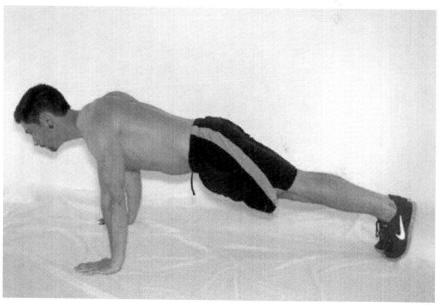

Pillar #2 (Intermediate) – Lower Body – Power Squats

This is a basic squat that is great for beginners, particularly if you have any knee issues. When you perform the squat try and keep you back as straight as possible at all times. One trick is to pretend that someone has just dropped an ice cube down your back. This is the kind of arch you will want to maintain in your back at all times. If you have difficulty keeping your balance at first try holding onto a chair. When you can perform 50 straight squats you are doing well.

1. Begin with your feet shoulder width apart and your arms straight out in front of you.
2. Keeping your back as straight as possible slowly start to bend your knees.
3. Your goal is to lower yourself to the point where your thighs are almost parallel to the floor. If you have knee issues simply go as low as you can.
4. Pause for a moment and then raise yourself back up. This counts as one rep.

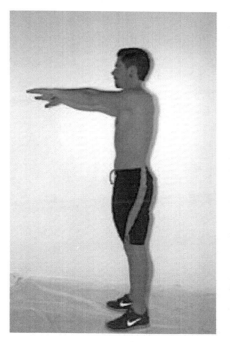 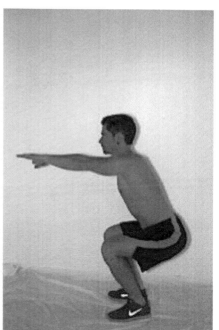

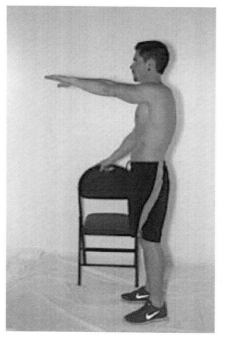 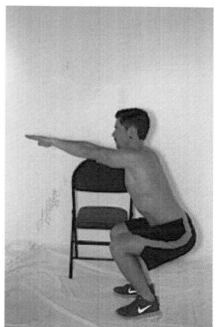

Pillar #3 (Intermediate) – Core – Seated Leg Lifts

This exercise will not only build strong lean abs but will tone your legs as well. When you can do 25 reps in a row you are doing well. Be warned though these are harder than they look.

1. Begin sitting on the ground with your legs straight and your arms behind you for support.
2. Keeping your legs straight lift them off the ground as high as they will go.
3. Keep your legs together through the movement.
4. Lower your legs to the ground. This constitutes one rep. To make the exercise harder don't let your feet hit the ground.

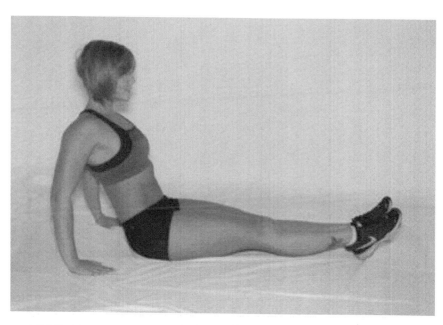

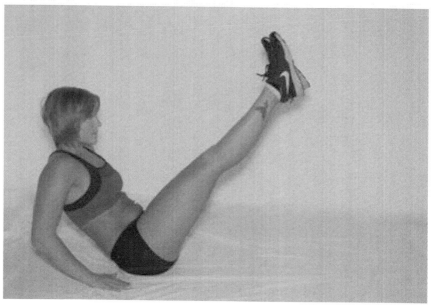

Pillar #4 (Intermediate) – Back Bending – Cobra Pushup

The cobra pushup is a variation of the cobra pose that is commonly done in yoga. Although it is called a pushup the primary muscles you want to use are those in your lower back. Your arms are only to be used for support.

1. Lie flat on your stomach with your hands by your chest.
2. Tighten your abs and breath in through your nose as you use your lower back muscles to lift your chest off the ground. Go as high as you are comfortable going. Use your arms only as support. The goal here is to strengthen your lower back.
3. At the highest point breathe out through your mouth as you hold this position for a count of 5.
4. Breathe in through your nose as you lower yourself to the ground.
5. Perform 15 repetitions.

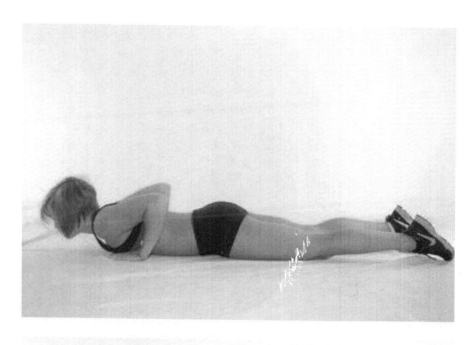

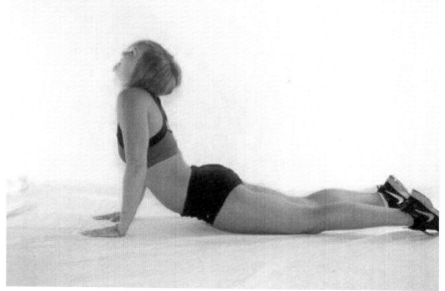

The Fantastic Four – Advanced Level

Perfection is not attainable, but if we chase perfection we can catch excellence. -Vince Lombardi

When you have reached this level you are doing fantastic and you are now fully prepared to experience all that bodyweight exercises have to offer. The exercises that make up the fantastic four at the advanced level are the most effective bodyweight exercises out there in my opinion. You could literally just do these four exercises three or four times a week and you'll be in fantastic shape. Do as many repetitions are you can handle at first. As you improve you will find the sky is literally the limit. For example, the Great Gama of India performed 500 Hindu squats everyday. You can do this as well, but it is not necessary. Most of us have no desire to be a world champion wrestler as most of us compete every day in a much more difficult competition, namely the game of life! In this case when you work up to 100 Hindu squats not only will you be in fantastic shape but also you'll be in better shape than 95% of the people you pass on the street. Good luck!

Pillar #1 (Advanced) – Upper Body – Hindu Pushups

Hindu Pushups originated in India where they are known as Dands. Indian wrestlers were famous for performing hundreds of these pushup daily and acquiring great strength and stamina as a result. Like all great bodyweight exercises Hindu Pushups work your entire body including your arms, back, chest and legs. It also massages your internal organs while increasing your flexibility. It also gives you a great cardio workout. You can do as many of these as you want but for most people a goal of 50 to 100 is desirable.

1. Begin with your butt in the air, your back straight and your hands shoulder width apart a few feet in front of you. Your legs should be straight as well with your feet two or three feet apart. This is the starting position. Take a deep breath through your nose.
2. Start lowering your chest to the ground by bending your elbows exhaling as you do so.
3. Continue to lower your hips to the ground so that your torso is almost parallel to the ground.
4. Push up and forward so that your arms are completely straight and your back is arched. Look up as far as you can while your exhale the last bit of air from your lungs.

5. Keeping your arms straight push your butt back into the air returning yourself to the starting position. Inhale through your nose as you do so.

Always remember that the entire motion should have a smooth and fluid aspect to it. Imagine that you are an ocean wave rolling onto the shore. Keep your mind focused and breathe deeply at all times.

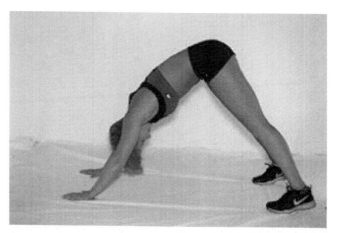

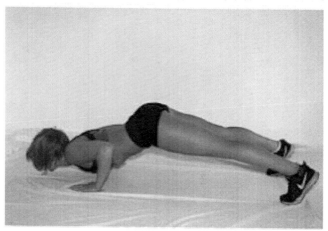

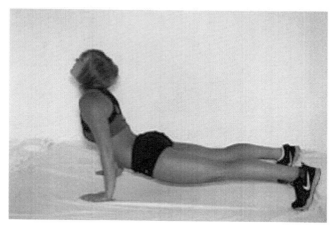

Pillar #2 (Advanced) – Lower Body – Hindu Squats

Hindu Squats are another fantastic bodyweight exercise, originating in India, which will simultaneously develop your legs and lungs. They will make you stronger and leaner while building tremendous muscular and cardiovascular endurance and help improve your balance. When you can do 50 Hindu Squats in a row you are doing well. For the average man or women doing 100 in a row is fantastic and you'll be in amazing shape as a result. If you want to shoot for superhuman aim to do 500 in under 15 minutes.

1. Being with your feet shoulder-width apart and your arms extended straight out in front of you parallel to the floor.
2. Breathe deeply through your nose as you clench your fists and pull them towards your chest.
3. Begin to lower your butt to the ground by bending your knees while keeping your back as straight as possible. Depending on your flexibility your heals may come off the ground or remain flat, either is fine. As you do so try to bring your hands behind your back. If you are taller and you find this difficult to do due to balance issues it is fine to keep your hands by your sides or in front of you.
4. As you lower yourself begin to exhale through your mouth.

5. Lower yourself as far as you can comfortably. This may mean that you can brush the ground with your hands but this is not necessary.
6. After you have reached the lowest point swing your arms forward forcefully as you explosive upwards by straightening your legs. You should exhale all of the remaining air from your lungs at this point.
7. Return to the starting point as in position one.

Like the Hindu Pushup the entire motion should be smooth and fluid like.

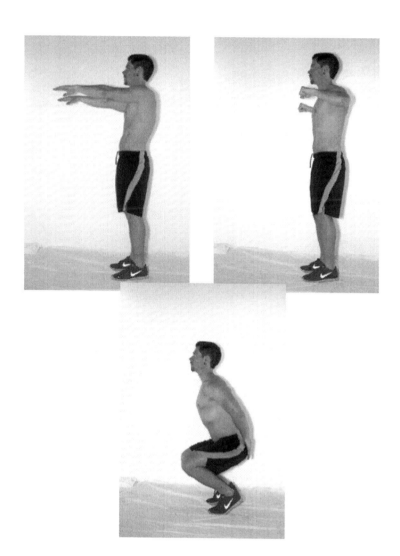

Pillar #3 (Advanced) – The Core – V-Ups

V-Ups are one of the most effective core exercises around and is a staple training tool of gymnasts and martial artists alike. Your goal is to imitate a jackknife closing and opening. When done correctly V-Ups will develop strength, balance and stabilization in both your upper and lower abdominal muscles.

1. Begin flat on your back with your legs straight and your arms over your head.
2. Exhale through your mouth as you raise your upper and lower body simultaneously.
3. Keep your arms and legs straight as you attempt to touch your hands to your feet. You should be balancing on your butt at this point.
4. Lower yourself back down to the starting position.
5. Do as many as you can until fatigued. 15 in a row is a good start. 50 in a row is fantastic.

Flexing your legs and pointing your toes during this exercise will help develop additional strength and shape in the legs as well.

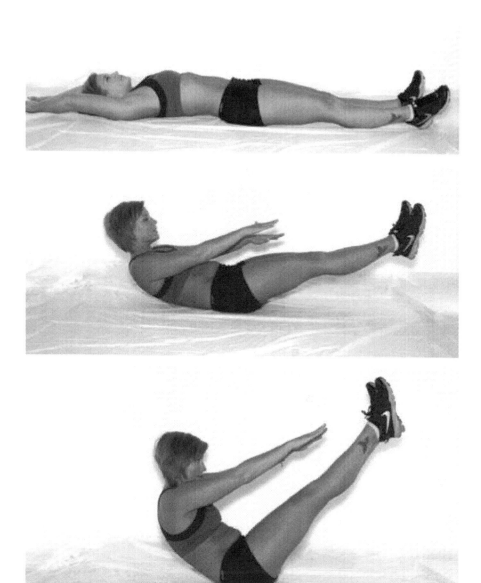

Pillar #4 (Advanced) – Back Bending – Back Bridge

There is no better exercise for strengthening and stretching the neck and back than the bridge. Sometimes called the wrestler's bridge this exercise will also strengthen your abs, butt and legs while simultaneously improving your circulation as well. I know how intimidating it looks at first glance but unless you have some kind of pre-existing medical condition I urge you to give it a try. It really is one of the best bodyweight exercises out there.

Warm Up

In order to get your neck and spine ready to perform the back bridge it is a good idea to warm up first by rocking back and forth. If you have never attempted to perform a full back bridge you might want to stick with this warm-up until your neck strengthens and you get used to the motion.

1. Lie down on your back on a soft mat or carpet.
2. Position your feet close to your butt. Place your hands face down by your shoulders.
3. Press up with your legs so that you arch your back while driving your body backwards.

4. Your weight should be supported by your feet, hands and the top of your forehead. Now rock back and forth so that you roll on your head. Your goal is to touch your nose to the floor before rocking back to a more neutral position.
5. When you can rock back and forth ten times touching your nose to the mat you are ready to move onto the back bridge.

Back Bridge

The only difference between the warm up and the full back bridge is that once you touch your nose to the mat you will want to hold this position for time. Your goal is to work up to holding this position for three minutes. Initially when you perform this exercise your heels will likely come off the ground when you arch your back. As you gain flexibility try to keep your feet flat on the ground. When you gain enough strength and confidence you can try performing the back bridge hands-free so long as your nose is touching the mat. It is very important to never hold your breath during this exercise. Breathe freely and deeply at all times.

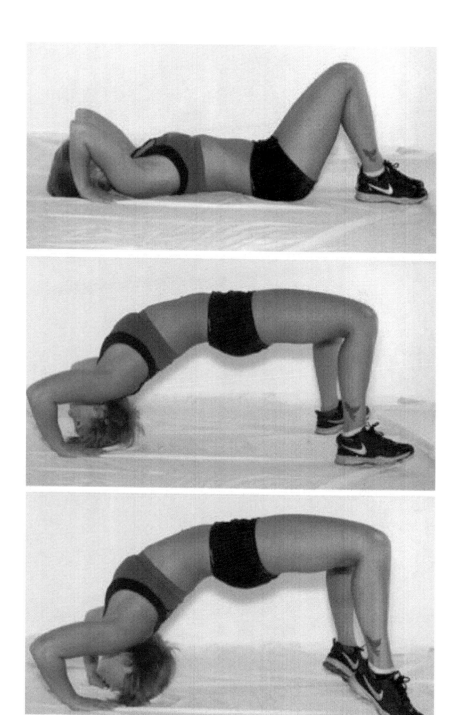

Supplementary Exercises

Never give up, for that is just the place and time that the tide will turn – Harriet Beecher Stowe

Once you feel you have mastered the four pillars of bodyweight fitness you can start to try these supplemental exercises for variety. You can either do these exercises in addition to the fantastic four foundation or replace one with another. However you do it, I recommend that your keep the foundation in place and always perform at least one exercise that involves working your upper body, lower body, core and a back bend.

The upcoming sections are organized by the four pillars. I have arranged them by putting the easier exercises first followed by those that are more challenging. I suggest that you begin with the easier exercises before moving onto the more advanced. Have fun and good luck.

Pillar #1 - Upper Body Exercises

*Love never fails; Character never quits; &
with patience & persistence; Dreams do come
true. - Pete Maravich*

Combo Pushups

This pushup is great for people who find full pushups too hard but knee pushups too easy.

1. Get in a pushup position on the floor with your ankles crossed and your knees bent.
2. Take a deep breath through your nose and then exhale through your mouth as you press yourself off the floor.
3. At the top of the movement uncross your ankles and straighten your legs. You should now be in a full pushup position.
4. Inhale through your nose and lower yourself to the ground.
5. Once you are on the floor re-cross your ankles and get back into the starting position. Repeat until fatigued.

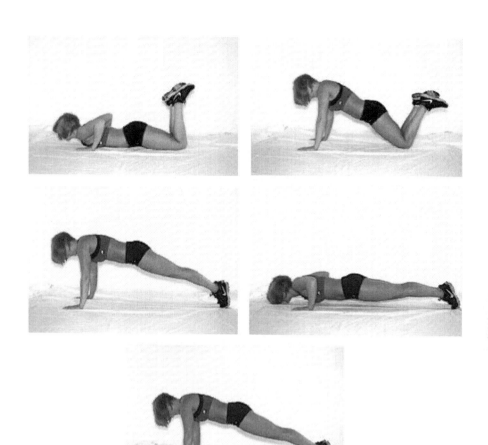

Walk Out Pushup

This exercise combines a pushup with a mini bear crawl and is perfect for indoor training.

1. Begin with your arms by your sides and your feet together.
2. Squat down and place your hands in front of you.
3. Crawl forward until you are in the classic pushup position.
4. Perform a single pushup.
5. Walk your hands backward and return to the crouch position.
6. Stand and repeat until fatigued.

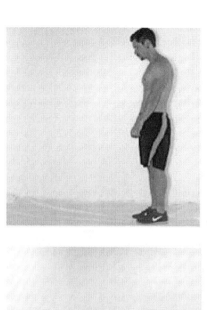
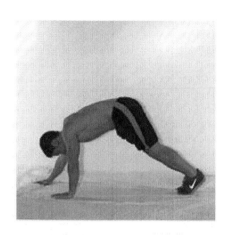
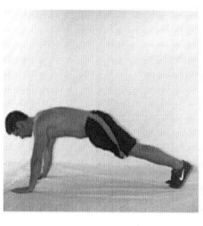
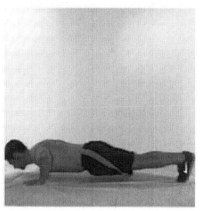
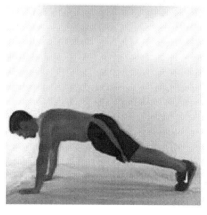
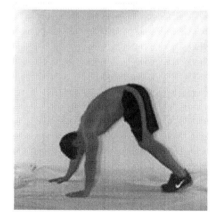

Pike Pushup

Pike pushups will really give you a sense of what it's like to work with your own bodyweight. They not only build tremendous arm and shoulder strength but will help tone your abs as well.

1. Assume the standard pushup position and then walk your hands backward until your body resembles an inverted "V".
2. The closer your hands are to your feet the harder the exercise will be.
3. Your arms and legs should be completely straight.
4. Inhale through your nose as you lower your head to the ground, exhale as you press back up.
5. Complete as many repetitions as you can.

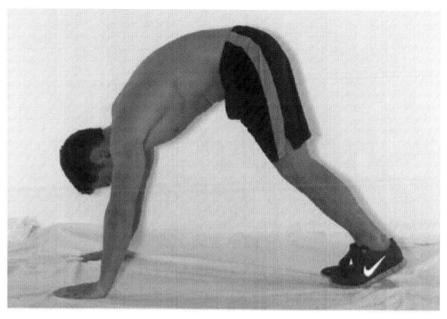

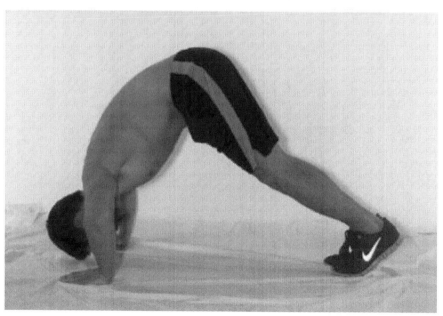

Reverse Handstand

A handstand is one of the best exercises you can do as it strengthen and tone your entire body. Your arms and shoulders will get most of the work but your abs will feel it as well. As a bonus this exercise will also help with your balance and will develop your kinesthetic body awareness. When you can hold a handstand for a minute you are doing great. When you can hold it for three minutes you are doing fantastic.

1. Begin in a pushup position with your feet against a solid wall.
2. Start walking backwards with your hands while you simultaneously walk up the wall with your feet. Go as far as you can while maintaining your balance.
3. From the handstand position breathe deeply and simply hold it as long as you can. Walk forward on your hands when you are finished. Be careful, as this exercise is harder than it looks.

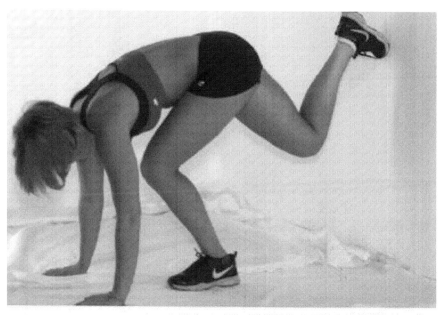

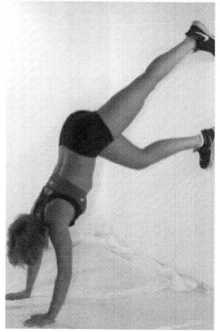
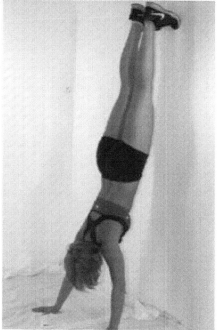

Elevated Pike Pushup

This is a more advanced version of the pike pushup. It is an excellent to perform if you are interested in building strength to perform a handstand pushup.

1. Begin by placing your feet on a stable elevated object like a chair with your hands on the floor in front of you.
2. Walk your hands backward so that your upper body is perpendicular to the ground.
3. Inhale through your nose as you lower your body towards the floor. Inhale through your mouth as you press yourself back up.
4. Do as many as you can until fatigued.

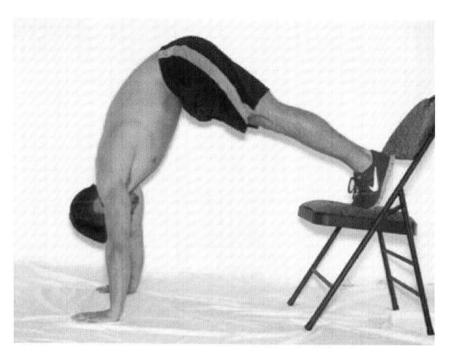

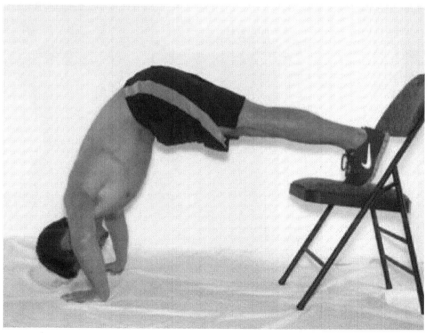

Atlas Pushups

It was none other than legendary fitness pioneer Charles Atlas who popularized this pushup variation. Performing the exercise with two sturdy chairs allows you to deeply work your chest muscles.

1. Begin by placing two chairs slightly more than shoulder width apart.
2. Place your hands on the chairs and assume a standard pushup position keeping your back straight and your abs tight.
3. Breathe in through your nose as you lower yourself as far as you can between the chairs. Exhale through your nose as you press yourself up.
4. Do as many as you can until you are fatigued. When you can do 25 in a row you are doing well. When you can do 100 you are approaching legendary status.

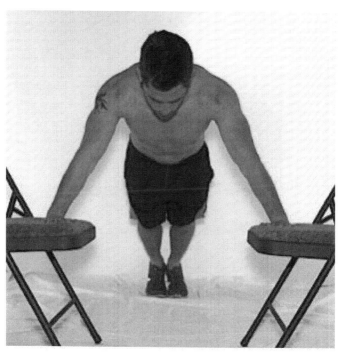

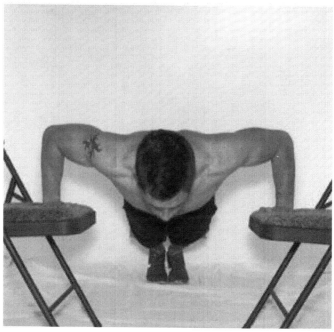

Reverse Pushups

Reverse pushups are what bodyweight fitness exercises are all about. Performing them will strengthen your shoulders, back and arms while toning your glutes and core. They will also increase the flexibility in your shoulders, back and abdominal region. It is simply a great bodyweight exercise to do.

1. Begin with your back on the floor and your feet close to your butt. Place your hands close to your shoulders with your palms flat on the ground.
2. Push your body off the floor as far as you can using your legs and arms. Aim to straighten your arms while you arch your back. Use your legs to drive your body backwards. Try and get your chest even with your arms.
3. Hold the highest position you can achieve for a count of three. At first this might mean only getting two inches off the ground. That's fine. Do what you can do.
4. Slowly lower yourself to the floor. You want your upper back to touch the floor first, not your head.
5. Do as many reps as you can until fatigued. When you can do ten in a row you are doing well.

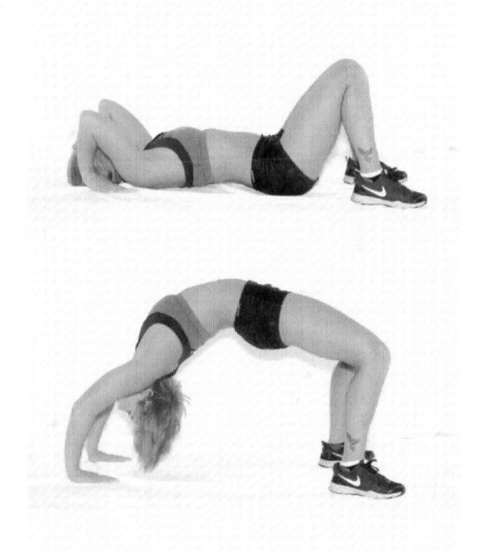

One Leg In The Air Pushups

This is a great exercise that will help you build the necessary strength to perform one-armed pushups.

1. Begin in the standard pushup position with your feet together and your hands shoulder width apart.
2. Breathe in through your nose as you shift your weight to your right shoulder by swinging the opposite leg towards it. Swivel your head in the opposite direction you are swinging your leg as you lower your body to the floor.
3. Your goal is to place as much weight on your right side so that your right arm and shoulder are doing most of the work.
4. Inhale through your mouth as you press your body back up to the starting position. Repeat the pushup on the opposite side.
5. Perform as many pushups as you can until fatigued.

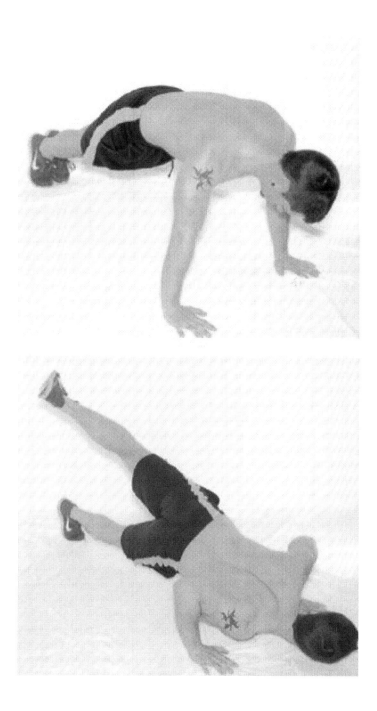

Handstand Pushups

In my opinion handstand pushups may well be the king of all upper body exercises. It is simply the best exercise I've found for building unreal shoulder and arm strength. To be able to push yourself up from a handstand position means you possess incredible upper body strength and upper body control.

1. Begin by placing your hands on the floor about 18 inches from a sturdy wall with your right knee under your chest.
2. Kick up into a handstand by kicking up with your left leg while pushing up with your right. Try to touch your feet to the wall as softly as you can.
3. Inhale through your nose as you slowly lower yourself as far as you can go.
4. Exhale through your mouth as you press yourself back up. If you cannot press yourself back up you have gone too far. Even if you only lower yourself a half an inch start there. Do what you can do to start with.
5. Do as many as you can until fatigued. When you can perform 10 in a row you are doing great.

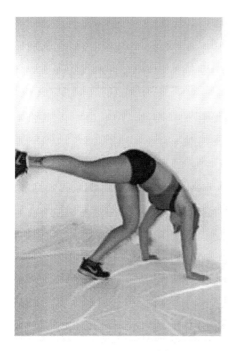 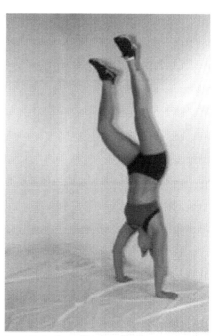

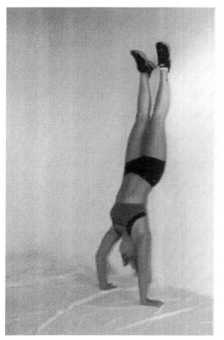 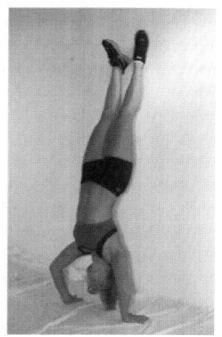

Pillar #2 - Lower Body Exercises

The greatest pleasure in life is doing what people say you cannot do - Walter Bagehot

Good Mornings

This exercise looks easy but it really works your glutes, hamstrings and lower back. When you bend forward keep your back arched. To help you with this imagine someone has dropped an ice cube down your back. That arch in your back is what you will want to strive to maintain when you bend forward. When you do this exercise properly you should feel a slight tension in the back of your legs.

1. Begin with your feet shoulder width apart and your hands behind your head.
2. Suck your stomach in and then bend forward at the waist.
3. You can bend your knees a little if needed but you should strive to keep you legs as straight as possible.
4. Return to the starting position. Try to do between ten and twenty at a time.

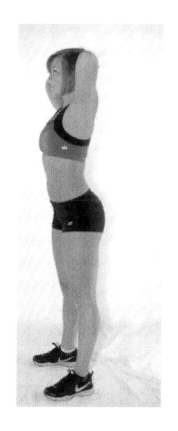 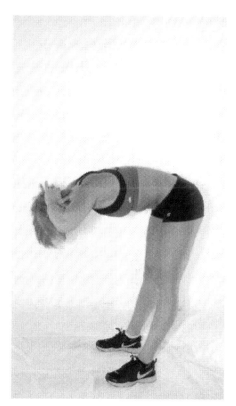

One Legged Bootstrappers

Working a single limb by itself is an incredibly effective training tool. The reason is that the body will allow a single limb to work harder by itself then if it is working with its partnered limb.

1. Begin in the "Up" position of a regular bootstrap except this time place your right foot on your left Achilles tendon. Your left heel should be flat on the ground.
2. Bend you left leg and squat down as far as you can go. Allow your left heel to come of the ground if needed.
3. Press you leg back up and repeat until fatigued.
4. Repeat this exercise with the opposite leg.

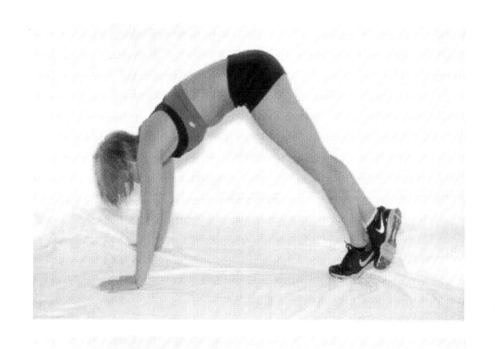

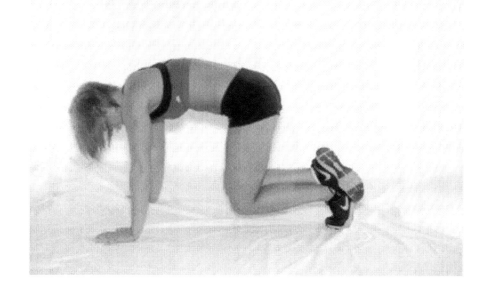

Lunges

Lunges are very effective in building shape, flexibility and strength in your legs while simultaneously improving your cardiovascular endurance and balance.

1. Begin standing with your legs shoulder width apart.
2. Lunge forward with your left leg. You will want to try and bend your left knee till it's at a 90-degree angle if possible. If you have knee issues simply bend it as far as you can.
3. Press back up with your left leg and return to the starting position.
4. Lunge forward with the right leg.
5. Repeat this sequence until fatigued. When you can perform 15 reps with each leg you are doing well.

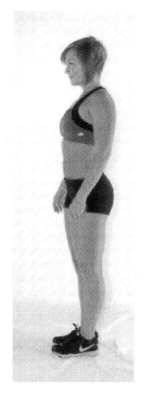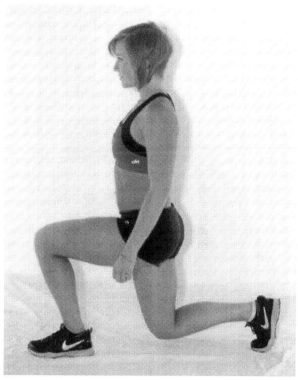

Sumo Squat

This exercise will not only build tremendous leg strength but also will also increase your flexibility in your inner thighs and groin. Make sure you always look straight ahead when you perform this exercise as this will help keep your back straight.

1. Begin with your heels slightly wider than shoulder width apart and your toes turned out to the sides as far as they can comfortably go.
2. Breathe in through your nose as you lower yourself to the ground. Go as far as you can comfortably go while keeping your back straight at all times. You should feel a gentle stretch in your hips, groin and lower back.
3. Exhale through your mouth as you raise your body back to the starting position.
4. Perform this movement slowly and deliberately for between 10 and 20 reps.

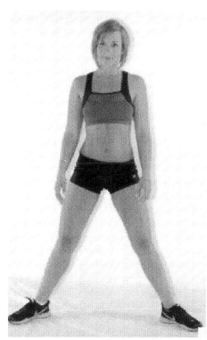

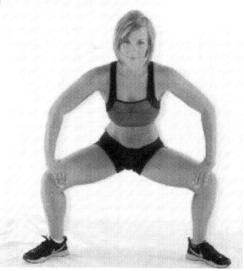

Wall Chair

This exercise is a staple for athletes who require tremendous leg strength such as skiers, speed skaters and hockey players. If you have knee issues and therefore have difficulty performing any kind of bodyweight squat this exercise is for you.

1. Begin by placing your back against a wall and your legs hip width apart.
2. Lower yourself so that your knees bend at a 90-degree angle, almost like you're sitting in an invisible chair. If you cannot hold this position at a 90-degree angle go as far as you can comfortably.
3. Press your feet into the ground, fold your arms in front of your chest and breathe deeply.
4. Relax and hold this position as long as you can. Make sure you don't give up at the first sign of fatigue.
5. When you can hold a wall chair for between two and three minutes you are doing well.

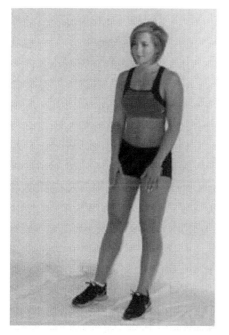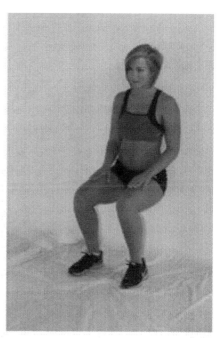

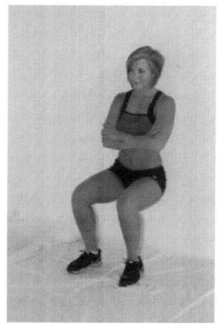

Ankle Raise

This exercise looks simple but is incredibly effective for strengthening your calves and ankles. It will also sculpt your thighs, glutes and abs while improving your balance and posture.

1. Begin with your ankles close together and your feet out at a 45-degree angle.
2. Lift your ankles off the ground so that you are standing on your toes while simultaneously squeezing your leg and glute muscles.
3. Lower yourself down to the starting position.
4. Your goal should be to do 20 repetitions in a row.

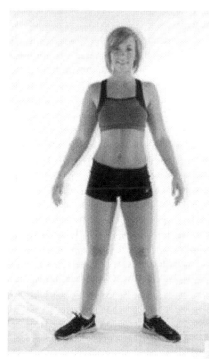

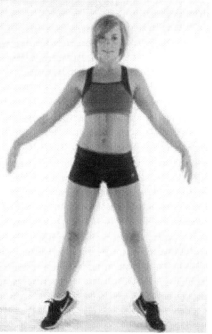

Quad Busters

This is another exercise that is actually far harder than it looks and will really work your hamstrings and quads. Make sure that you keep your abdominal muscles tight throughout this exercise in order to protect your lower back.

1. Begin with your legs together and then bend forward so that you can grab your ankles. Bend your knees as much as you need to in order to bend forward comfortably. However, try to keep you legs as straight as possible.
2. Take a deep breath through your nose so that you completely fill your lungs.
3. As you exhale through your mouth bend your knees until your butt touches your ankles. If you are not flexible enough to reach this far simply bend as far as you can go.
4. Breathe in through your nose as you straighten your legs back to the starting position.
5. Do as many as you can until fatigued. When you can to 20 in a row you are doing well.

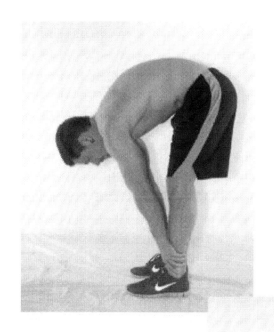

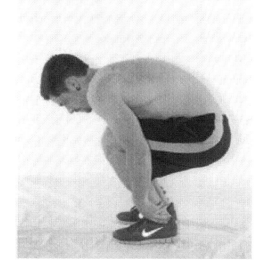

Flamingo Jumps

This exercise will shape your legs while building strength, balance and agility.

1. Begin standing on your right leg with your left leg lifted up at a 90-degree angle in front of you. Straighten your arms out by your side for balance.
2. Bend your right knee.
3. Jump as high as you can using just your right leg. The jump should be explosive.
4. Land on your right leg and regain your balance.
5. Perform 10 jumps per leg.

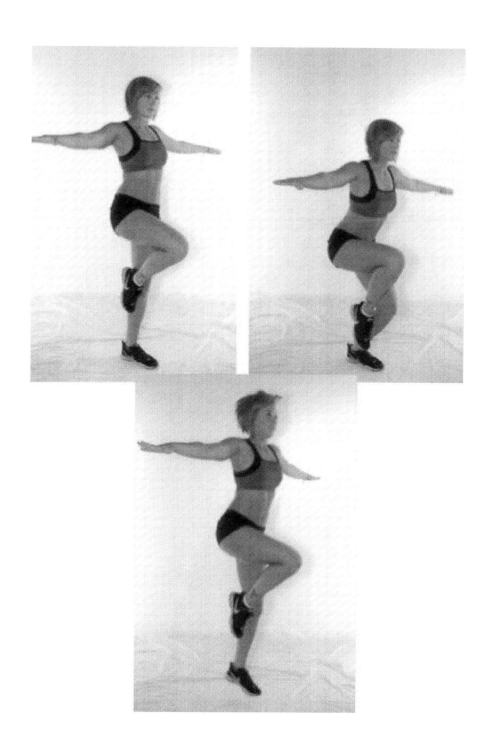

Genie Jumps

Performing these jumps builds explosive strength in the legs while simultaneously building your cardiovascular endurance.

1. Begin with your feet wider than your hips and your arms folded across your chest.
2. Inhale deeply through your nose as you squat down slightly.
3. Exhale through your mouth as you jump as high as you can while bringing your legs together.
4. Widen your feet as you come down so that you land in the starting position.
5. Do as many as you can until fatigued. When you can do 50 in a row you are doing well.

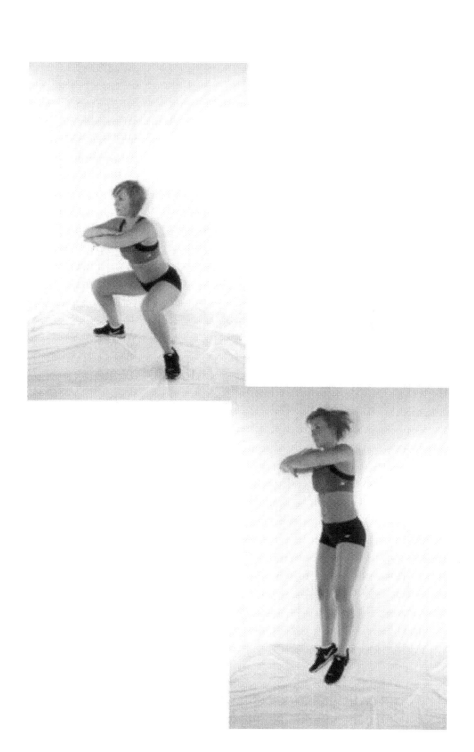

One Legged Squats

One-legged squats are probably the greatest exercise you can do to build incredible strength in your legs and glutes. You don't have to do too many of them to get the full benefits of this exercise. When you are first starting I suggest you perform it with a chair for balance as shown. As you get stronger and your balance improves you will want to try it without the chair.

1. Begin by standing on one leg while lifting your other leg straight in front of you. Hold onto something like a chair in order to help you with your balance if needed.
2. Keeping your head up and your back straight inhale through your nose and start to slowly lower your body to the ground. Go as far as you can. This might mean only a few inches at first, which is fine. Stop as soon as you feel any discomfort in the knee.
3. Keep you stomach tight at all times.
4. Squat back up by exhaling through your mouth and pressing your foot hard into the ground.
5. Do as many as you can until fatigued. When you can perform 10 repetitions on each leg you are doing well.

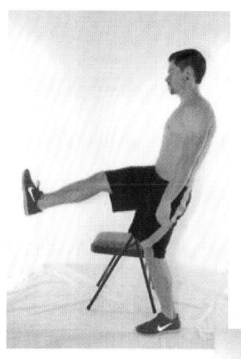

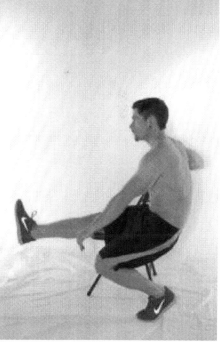

Pillar #3 – The Core

You are never too old to set another goal or to dream a new dream – C.S. Lewis

Tai Chi Waist Turner

Do not be misled by how simple this exercise appears. Although it is easy to do it will massage your internal organs, increase the flexibility in your spine and help reduce your waistline. It is an excellent exercise to do first thing in the morning. I would recommend performing 50 to 100 repetitions.

1. Begin with your feet shoulder width apart and your arms hanging loosely by your sides.
2. Keep your feet planted as you begin to twist your entire spine from side to side. As you do so allow the centrifugal force you are generating to move your arms freely.
3. Each time you have twisted as far as you're comfortably can to one side allow your hands to gently slap you in the kidneys. This will give them a gentle massage.

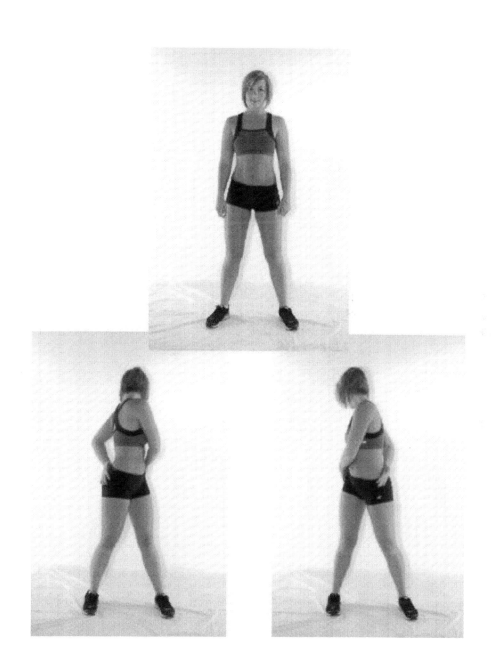

Side Bends

This exercise excels at strengthening and stretching your waist.

1. Begin by standing with your feet together and one arm in the air. This is the starting position.
2. Take a deep breath through your nose.
3. As you exhale through your mouth bend at the waist as far as you can go to the opposite side of your raised arm.
4. Inhale through your nose as you raise your body slightly by about five degrees. You are only moving enough to work the muscles on the side of your waist. You are not returning to the starting position.
5. Repeat this slight back and forth movement 50 to 100 times.
6. Repeat this exercise on the opposite side of your body.

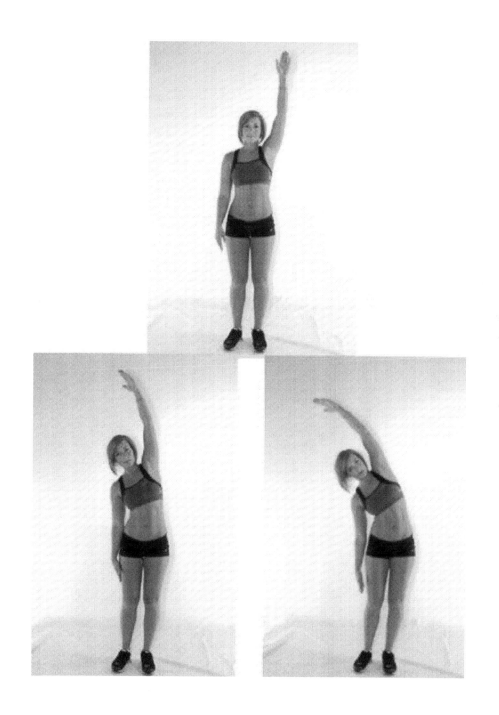

Leg Lifts

Performed correctly leg lifts will strengthen and tone your lower abs. When performing this exercise always focus on feeling your abs working as opposed to using your hips. A variation is to perform this exercise with your head raised off the ground as this will help strengthen your neck.

1. Begin by lying on your back with your hands under your butt.
2. Raise your legs off the ground until they are at a 45 to 90 degree angle.
3. During the entire movement try to flex your legs straight while keeping your toes pointed. Try to keep your knees straight. Doing this will lengthen and tone your leg muscles.
4. Hold the "Up" position for 2 seconds before lowering your legs to just above the floor in a controlled manner.
5. Do until fatigued. When you can do 20 repetitions in a row you are doing well.

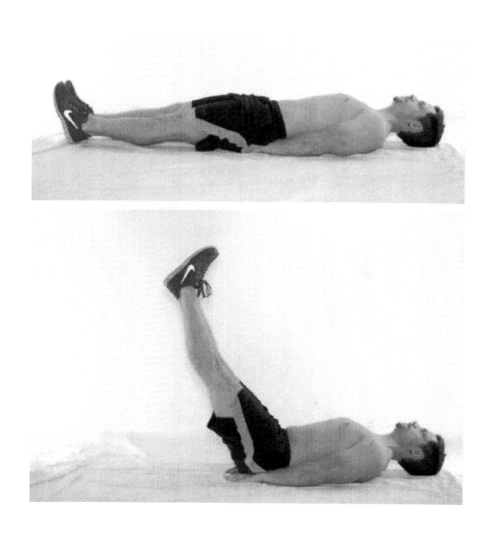

Sideward Leg Lifts

Sideward leg lifts will help you develop flexibility and strength in your hips and thighs.

1. Begin by lying on your side with your legs together.
2. Lift both legs off the ground at the same time. Inhale through your nose as you lift them up, exhale as you lower them to the floor.
3. Repeat until fatigued and then switch sides.

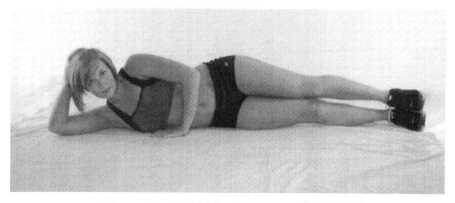

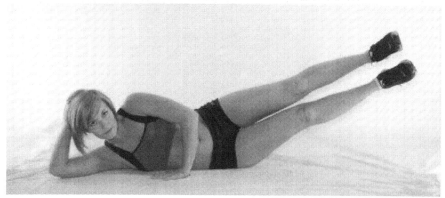

The Table Maker

This exercise will work your core while building strength and flexibility in your spine, back, triceps, shoulders, hips and buttocks.

1. Begin by sitting on the floor with your back straight and your legs straight out in front of you. Place your palms beside your hips.
2. Inhale through your nose as you push your body forward until the soles of your feet are flat on the ground. Arch your hips and back and let your head fall backward.
3. Squeeze your back and abs tightly as you straighten your back as much as you can. Your goal is to make a table out of your body with your arms and legs at a 90-degree angle to your core.
4. Hold the table position for a beat and then lower yourself back to the starting position.
5. Repeat until fatigued. When you can perform between 10 and 20 repetitions of this exercise you are doing well.

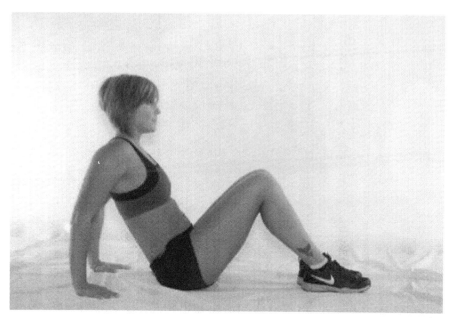

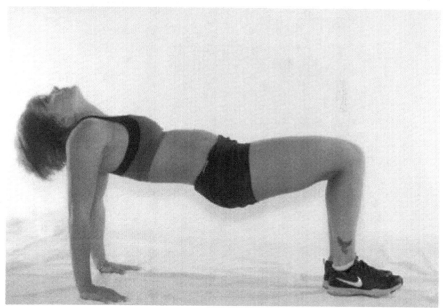

No Momentum Sit-Ups

This exercise is performed slowly and deliberately, which makes it almost impossible to cheat. Your goal is to imitate a zombie or a vampire rising from the grave. It is this slow motion that will really strengthen your abdominals, lower back and hip flexors.

1. Begin by lying on the floor with your arms by your sides.
2. Slowly start to raise your upper body off the ground using your abdominal muscles only. Your heels and legs should never come off the floor.
3. Continue to rise until your upper body is perpendicular to the floor.
4. Reverse direction and lower your upper body to the ground. Make sure you go slowly here as well as you want to work your muscles in both directions.
5. Perform as many as you can until fatigued.

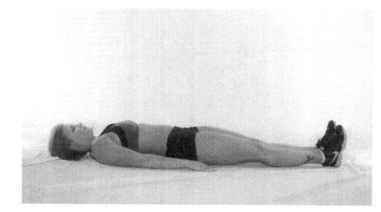

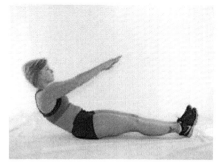
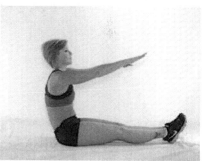

Toes Behind Head Leg Lifts

This is a great exercise for your abdominals that will also increase the flexibility of your back and legs. It will also help increase your circulation, massage your internal organs and aid in the digestive process.

1. Begin by lying flat on your back with your hands by your side and your legs straight.
2. Keeping your legs straight at all times point your toes and lift them all the way over your head.
3. Touch your toes to the ground behind you.
4. Return your legs back to the starting position.
5. Do as many repetitions as you can until fatigued.

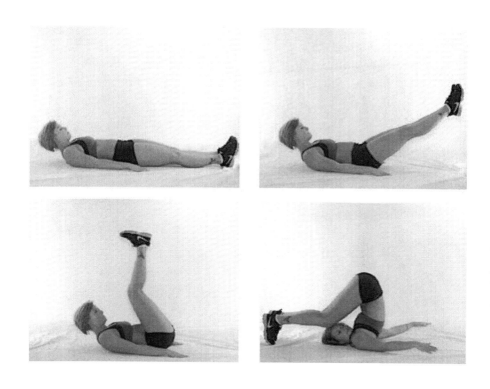

Leg Scissors

Leg scissors will not only work you abdominals but will hit your inner and outer thighs as well as your hip flexors.

1. Begin by lying flat on your back with your legs straight and your arms by your side.
2. Tuck your chin into your chest as you simultaneously lift both legs about 6 inches off the floor. Your legs can either be straight or slightly bent.
3. Inhale through your nose as you open your legs wide.
4. Exhale through your mouth as you reverse direction and cross your legs.
5. Continue until fatigued. When you can do between 25 and 50 repetitions you are doing well.
6. Remember to alternate the leg that goes under and over on each repetition.

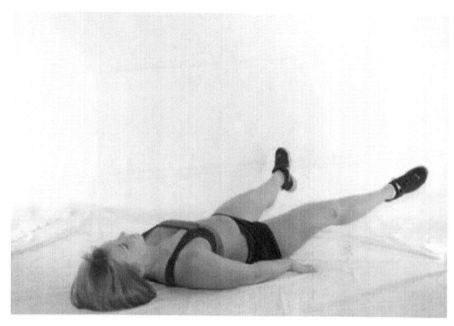

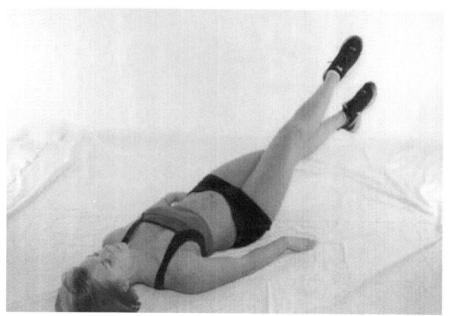

Russian Twists

This exercise really hits your entire core region as both your upper and lower body are off the ground. The twisting motion will really strengthen your obliques as well as help with the suppleness of your spine.

1. Begin by sitting up on the ground with your feet raised in front of you.
2. Fold your arms across your chest and then begin to twist at your torso from left to right.
3. Make sure you keep your feet off the ground at all times.
4. Do as many twists as you can until fatigued.

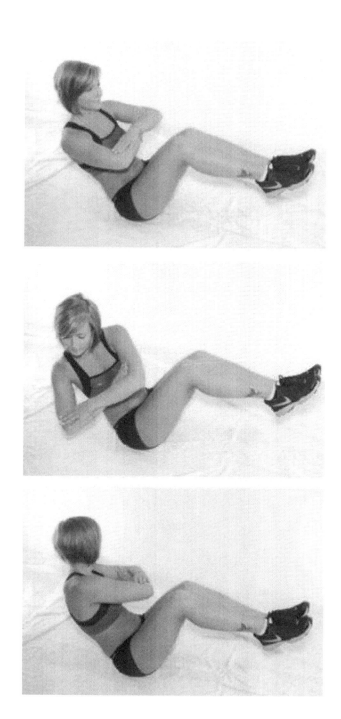

Headstand Leg Tuck

Headstands are a terrific exercise as the act of balancing works your entire body, especially your core.

1. Begin by placing a towel or pillow in front of a sturdy wall if you are on a hard surface.
2. Squat down and place your forehead in the palm of your hands. Let your elbows come out so that they form a triangle on the floor with your head.
3. Place your knees on your elbows and slowly lift your feet off the ground.
4. Exhale through your mouth as you slowly straighten your legs in a controlled fashion.
5. Keep your legs straight for a second and then inhale through your nose as you lower your legs while maintaining the headstand.
6. Repeat this exercise until fatigued. When you can do 10 in a row you are doing well.

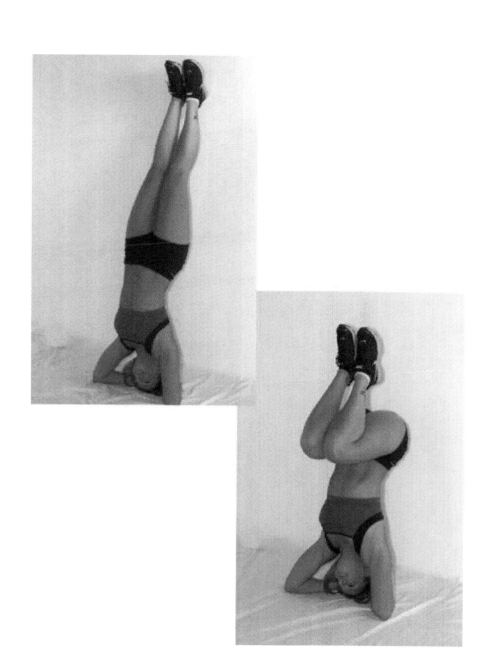

Pillar #4 – Back Bending Exercises

Each one of us has a fire in our heart for something. It's our goal in life to find it and to keep it lit – Mary Lou Retton

Kneeling Back Arch

This exercise not only works your back but your abs and butt as well.

1. Kneel on the floor with your arms and thighs at a 90-degree angle to your body.
2. Exhale through your mouth as you look up while allowing your back to curve downward. Hold this position for a count of 10.
3. Inhale through your mouth as you allow your head to fall forward while arching your back upward. Hold for another count of 10.
4. Perform this movement slowly and deliberately while ensuring that your weight is evenly distributed between your knees and hands.
5. Repeat this movement 10 times.

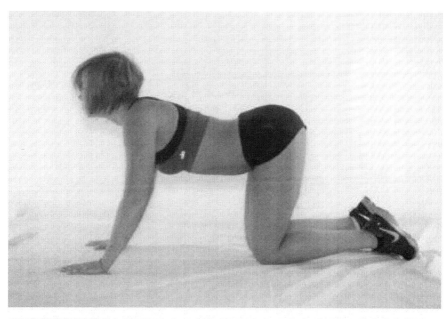

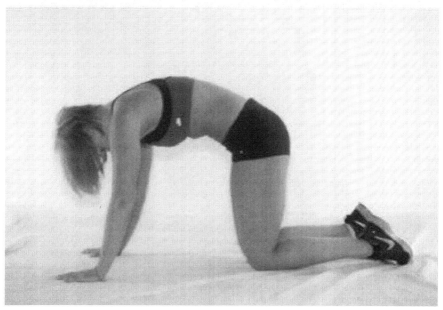

131

Reverse Leg Lifts

This exercise stretches and strengthens your lower back at the same time while working your abdominals and glutes, as well. When you lift your legs it is very important to keep you nose on the floor in order to protect your lower back.

1. Begin by lying flat on the floor face down with your arms stretched forward.
2. Inhale through your nose and use your back muscles to lift both of your legs at the same time. Try and hold this position for a count of 5.
3. Exhale through your mouth and slowly lower you legs to the floor.
4. Repeat this movement 10 times.

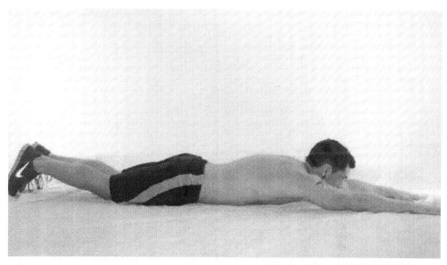

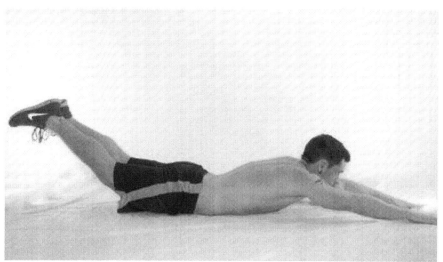

Torso Lifts

Torso lifts are the opposite of the reverse leg lifts although they still work your back and abdominals.

1. Lie face down on the floor with your arms stretched forward.
2. Inhale through your nose filling your lungs.
3. Exhale through your mouth as you lift your arms, chest and abdominals as high as can. Keep your legs on the ground at all times while squeezing your butt to protect your lower back. Hold this position for a count of 5.
4. Lower yourself to the floor and inhale through your nose.
5. Repeat this exercise 10 times or until fatigued.

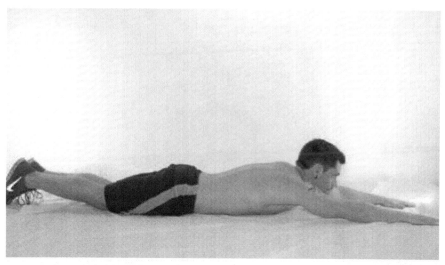

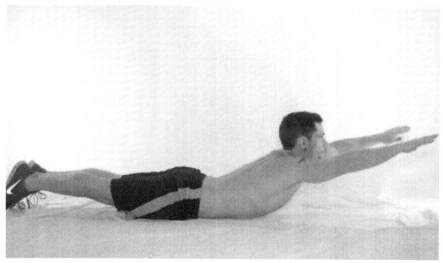

Swimmers

This exercise is fantastic for strengthening your back while simultaneously sculpting your glutes.

1. Begin by lying flat down on your stomach with your arms in front of you.
2. Slowly raise your right leg and your left arm as high as possible.
3. Hold this position at its highest point for 3 seconds.
4. Lower your arm and leg to the ground and then repeat with your opposite arm and leg.
5. Switch back and forth in this manner until fatigued. When you can do 10 in a row you are doing well.

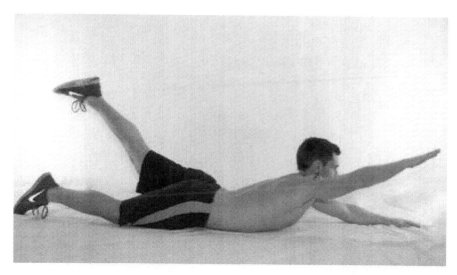

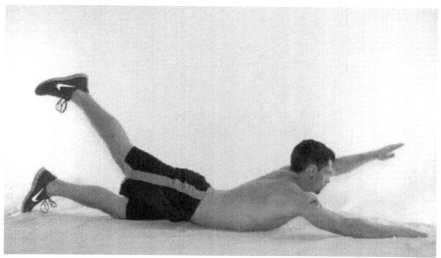

Arch Ups

This exercise combines the torso lift and reverse leg exercises. It is excellent for developing a strong back, shoulders, legs and glutes while increasing your flexibility.

1. Begin by lying on your stomach with your arms shoulder width apart and your legs together.
2. Stretch your body lengthwise.
3. Tighten your butt and abdominal muscles as you arch your back, lifting your arms and legs off the ground as you do so.
4. When you've arched your back as far as it will go hold this position for a count of two while keeping your arms by your ears. Your body should be shaped liked the bottom of a rocker on a rocking chair.
5. Lower yourself back to the starting position.
6. Do as many as you can until fatigued. When you can do 25 in a row you are doing well.

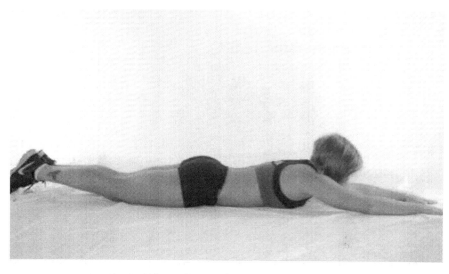

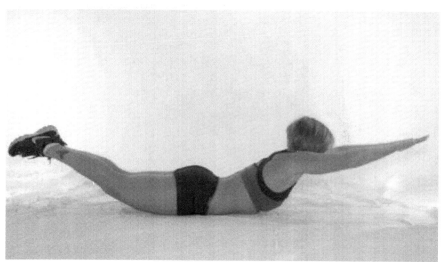

Floor Bow Posture

This posture is commonly practiced in yoga. It is fantastic at increasing the flexibility of your spine while stretching and strengthening the muscles as well. When I perform the floor bow I generally get the best results doing it twice. You can do more if you feel your back needs it.

1. Begin by lying flat on your stomach.
2. Grab your ankles from the outside with either hand.
3. Use your legs to kick up and backward. All of the force should be generated by your legs, not your arms. Your arms should be like ropes. They are attached to your ankles, but they are not generating any pulling force themselves.
4. If you are able to try to look at the ceiling by bending your neck backwards. If your neck is stiff simply bend it backwards as far as you can.
5. Hold this position while taking five slow, deep breaths.

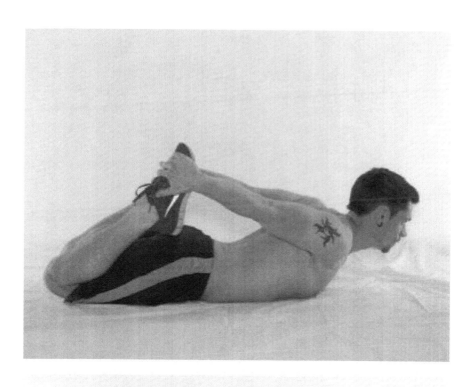

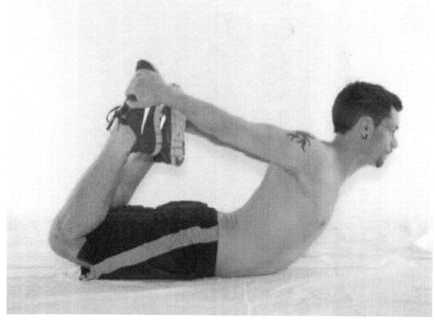

Gymnastic Bridge

The gymnastic bridge is a full body exercise that will build strength and flexibility in your shoulders, back, legs and abdominals. It is also a fantastic back bending exercise, which is why I've included it here. If you cannot get into the gymnastic bridge with your arms extended simply press up as far as you can go. With time and practice you will get stronger and you will still gain tremendous benefit by trying.

1. Begin by lying flat on your back with your legs bent and your palms by your shoulders.
2. Push off with your hands and legs, arching your back into the bridge.
3. Squeeze your butt and try to stretch your stomach as much as possible while using your legs to drive your chest forward.
4. Breathe slowly and deeply.
5. Try to hold this position for as long as you can. When you can hold it for a minute you are doing well. When you can hold it for 3 minutes you are doing fantastic.

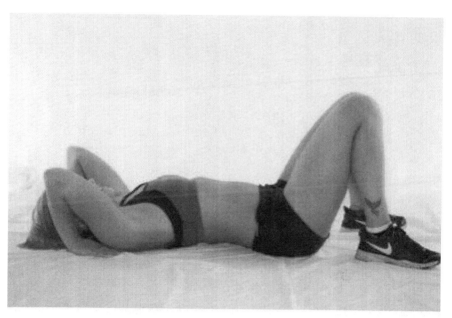

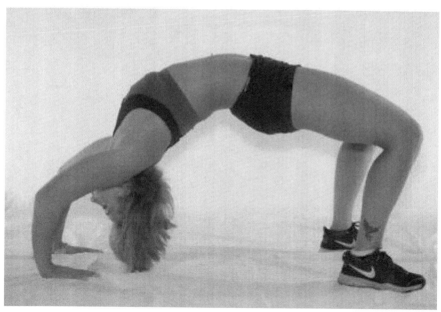

One Leg Gymnastic Bridge

Like its two-legged cousin this exercise will sculpt and strengthen your entire body. The raised leg however will really force you to maintain your balance, which will really work your core muscles. You should only attempt this exercise once your have mastered the gymnastic bridge.

1. Begin by getting into a good gymnastic bridge with your arms extended and chest forward.
2. Lift your right leg up as far as you can. Try and keep it as straight as possible.
3. Squeeze your butt and tighten your abdominal muscles.
4. Hold this position for as long as you can while breathing deeply.
5. Switch legs and repeat.

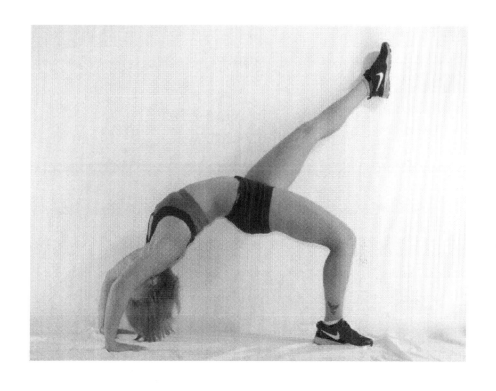

Nutritional Advice

*Our food should be our medicine and our
medicine should be our food. —Hippocrates*

This is a book about proper exercise, not
proper eating. Nonetheless, I do feel the need
to comment on the absolute requirement for
you to eat a healthy diet. There is an old fitness
saying that states you get stronger in the gym,
but you get lean in the kitchen. This is the
truth. You can perform the absolute best
bodyweight fitness fat burning workouts in the
world and not get lean if you don't follow a
clean, healthy diet. If you think it's possible to
get lean with exercise alone without watching
what you eat, think again.

What do I mean when I say you should strive
to eat a clean, healthy diet? By this, I mean,
you want to try and consume food that has not
been overly processed by man. Avoid foods
when possible that come in bags, boxes or
wrappers. The reason for this is simple: the
more food is processed by man, the
unhealthier and more fattening it becomes.

Consider the example of the potato. The
simplest method to prepare a potato is to cook
it in its own skin. When cooked this way, a
potato will contain roughly 145 calories and be
packed with vitamins and minerals and is 70%
water. What happens when you process this
same potato and you turn it into 10 French
Fries? For one, the calorie content will increase
to 214 calories, mostly in the form of fat. The
vitamin and mineral content is leeched out and

the water percentage is cut in half. Now, take that same potato and transform it into its most processed form, namely 20 potato chips. The calorie count is now 228 and very little healthy vitamins and minerals remain. What's more, a typical potato chip is only 2% water.

From this small example you can clearly see the negative effect that overly processing foods can have. What's worse is that while most people can limit themselves to one potato, who can only eat 10 French Fries or 20 potato chips? Most people are going to eat far more than that in one sitting with no difficulty at all.

Think of the animals in nature. Obviously all of the food they eat is completely unprocessed. Have you ever seen a fat fox? This doesn't mean you need to follow a raw food diet or anything like that (although some people would advocate it). However, you should be aware of what you are putting in your body. One suggestion I do have is to keep a food journal in which you record everything you eat. If, after exercising for a month or so, you are not losing weight as quickly as you'd like then take a look at your food journal. What junk are you still eating? What can you give up? Making small changes here can lead to big weight changes later. Just remember, you are always better off eating an apple than a piece of apple pie.

Are Bodyweight Squats Safe?

One question I often get regarding bodyweight squats is from people who question how safe they are. There is a feeling out there that some squats, like Hindu squats, are dangerous because your knees go over your toes and this will "shear the knee". Is there any truth to this argument? I don't think there is. Here's why.

In my opinion, squatting is a natural movement that human beings have adapted to. For thousands of years, human beings, without the benefit of furniture, have squatted in order to rest and perform a variety of activities. People still do this in large parts of Asia, for example. If sitting with your knees over your toes for long periods were dangerous, you would think that there would be an epidemic of knee-related issues in Asia. That this is not the case, indicates to me, that there is not much of a case to be made for the "shearing the knee" theory.

Another example is one of the main advocates of the Hindu squat, namely the Great Gama of India. Gama was a professional wrestler at the turn of the last century when professional wrestling was a real sport. He was known to perform between 500 and 1000 Hindu squats, or Dands, a day. There is no record of him having any kind of knee problems. In fact, it is quite the opposite. He was known as one of the strongest and best-conditioned athletes of his day and he never suffered from any knee problems.

Furthermore, I have looked and have yet to find one scientific study that makes the case for "knee shearing". If I'm wrong, by all means, please forward the information to me. However, I simply haven't seen it.

I suspect the concern with "knee shearing" is that most people are extremely protective of their knees as it is such a delicate joint. Bikram Choudhury, of Bikram Yoga fame, has a saying, "You can mess with the gods, you can mess with me, but don't mess with your knees." Once you have damaged your knees, it is extremely difficult to heal them. It is a good idea to be careful with your knees in all activities; however worrying about knee shearing isn't one of them.

When you start performing deep knee bends of any kind, it is not unusual to experience some discomfort (not pain, discomfort). This is just your body adjusting to your new physical regime and it will take some time to strengthen the tendons and ligaments around the knees, not to mention the muscles. This process usually takes about four weeks.

Having said that, you know your body better than anyone else. If you feel any kind of pain use your brain and modify the exercise as you see fit. In my case, the cartilage in my left knee is severely worn due to a lifetime of running and getting injured playing a variety of sports before I discovered bodyweight workouts. As a result, when I perform a squat I don't go as deeply as someone with a healthy knee might. Use your common sense and you'll be fine.

Notes On The Back Bridge

Of all the bodyweight exercises in this book, the exercise that most people approach with the most fear and trepidation is the back bridge. I understand this fear completely as I had it myself at one point as the exercise itself is so unusual. Some people even avoid trying the back bridge as it is so strange. This is a shame as the back bridge is probably the best exercise you can do to build real strength and flexibility along the entire neck and spine.

Most people's fear of the back bridge is rooted in the fear of how the neck is bent and the pressure that is potentially applied to it. So long as you have no prior neck injuries (as always, check with your doctor before beginning ANY exercise program), this shouldn't concern you. If you are like most people, your neck is likely weak as you probably never exercise it. However, this is a reason for exercising your neck with the back bridge, not avoiding it.

Have you ever wondered why some elderly people acquire such a stooped posture? It typically begins with having a weak neck. The head is very heavy and if the neck is weak, it will start to droop forward. As time passes, the head will then pull the shoulders (and eventually the upper spine forward, as well) which results in a hunched back. Bending backward, while strengthening the neck and spine, is the best preventive medicine for this.

Another concern is that too much pressure is applied to the neck during the back bridge.

This shouldn't be a concern as you can regulate the pressure with your hands. As well, not all of the pressure is born by the neck, even when you perform a hands-free back bridge. A properly performed back bridge will strengthen your back, thighs, hips and buttocks along with your neck. How can this be if all the pressure is born by the neck? Clearly it isn't when it is done properly.

Another concern I hear is that the back bridge somehow "compresses" the spine and neck, which is not desirable. This doesn't make any sense. If you bend forward are you stretching your back? Of course you are. Why should it be any different if you bend your back backward? Back bends stretch and elongate the spine and neck. When an archer pulls back the string on a bow, is he compressing or stretching the bow? I think the answer is obvious.

The first time you try bridging, it will likely feel extremely awkward and unnatural. This is to be expected as you likely have never done it before. I remember the first back bridge I attempted. I could barely hold it and my spine made noises like tiny twigs were cracking. I was stiff. However, my back felt so much better afterwards so I kept at it and there is no doubt that my spine is stronger and healthier as a result. As with the bodyweight squats, I urge you to take it slow and listen to your body. A healthy spine equals a healthy life and there is no better exercise for a healthy spine than bridging.

FAQ

Will engaging in a bodyweight fitness program such as this one help me stay young?

Without question. Aging is a part of life and every one of us gets a little older everyday. However, I am of the firm belief that 90% of the physical decline we as human beings associate with aging has to do with inactivity and not with the passage of time itself. Think of animals in the wild. If you encounter an old bear in the woods you still have to be careful as it is still a formidable animal. It is not walking around with a walker or living in a wheel chair. The primary reason an old bear is so much healthier than most old people is that the bear is forced to keep exercising in order to survive whereas most people simply stop doing anything and are physical wrecks before the age of 30. Use it or lose it, as they say.

Another point I want to emphasize is the importance of maintaining fast twitch muscle fibers over time. Remember, fast twitch muscle fibers are what you use for fast paced, athletic movements. They are larger and more powerful than their slow twitch counterparts. Put another way, fast twitch fibers are the muscles of youth. When you see an old person who appears to be thin and frail the primary difference between them and you is that they have lost through inaction almost all of their fast twitch fibers. This is a similar effect to what you see when you compare the physiques of marathon runners to sprinters. The marathon runners' look smaller, weaker and older than their sprinting counterparts because their training doesn't involve working their fast twitch fibers. When muscles aren't worked, you lose them. The bottom line is that if you want to stay young you need to work those fast twitch muscle fibers. Natural bodyweight exercises are the best way to do this.

Should I exercise everyday?

My feeling is that you should try to at least a little something everyday. Do you have a shower everyday? Do you brush your teeth everyday? Animals in nature exercise everyday and they are obviously far healthier than any human being. Every workout you do doesn't have to be a killer. Even doing a little can have tremendous benefits. Personally I love to exercise first thing in the morning as it warms up my body and helps prepare it for the day. Now having said that we are all busy and sometimes time simply doesn't permit. So long as you're exercising three or four times a week you'll make great progress.

I've noticed there aren't any kinds of pulling exercises in your program. Why is this?

I have nothing against pulling exercises like chin-ups, for example. It is just that they typically require some form of equipment like a chin-up bar and I like to perform exercises that require no equipment at all. I've also found that they are not as important as a lot of people think. If you doubt this try this experiment. Record how many chin-ups you can do today and then start working on your handstand pushups. When you can do 15 handstand pushups in a row go back and try the chin-ups again. I think you'll be amazed at how much better you do. Again though I want to emphasize that I have nothing against pulling type exercises. If you do them now and enjoy them then by all means keep at it.

Why are people who perform bodyweight exercises so much stronger than those that lift weights exclusively?

I've often wondered about this myself. Like I stated previously a gymnast can easily throw around weights like nobody's business but a weight lifter will not be able to do the simplest bodyweight movements that the gymnast performs. A large part of the reason is that all bodyweight exercises force your muscles to work together as nature intended. Another reason is that bodyweight workouts force you to maintain balance at all times which works your muscles in different ways. Whatever the reason though if you want to be truly strong and not just gym strong bodyweight exercises are the way to go.

I like to lift weights. Can I still do this?

If you like lifting weights feel free. I know some people who lift weights three days a week and perform bodyweight exercises on their off days. I don't feel that lifting weights is necessary but if you enjoy doing it then keep doing it. Some people approach fitness almost like it is a religion and to try something different is to break the faith. I'm not that way at all. I only do bodyweight exercises but if you want to do something a little bit differently I won't stop you. I know a lot of people who lift weights because they like to sculpt their body in a certain way. There is nothing wrong with this it just isn't for me. Do what works for you.

As I travel a lot I spend a lot of time in hotel rooms. Can I perform these workouts in my hotel room?

Absolutely. In fact, these exercises are almost made for you. As they need no special equipment bodyweight exercise can be done anywhere at anytime, including on vacation and in hotel rooms.

I love the results I'm getting by doing the fantastic four. Can I just stick with this?

If you were to only do some version of the fantastic four three or four times a week, you'll be in better shape than 95% of the people out there. It really depends on your goals. If you simply want to be in great shape so that you can enjoy life then the fantastic four is all you need. If, on the other hand, you are training for a specific athletic endeavor, you may want to add more. For most people, though, the fantastic four is enough by itself.

My knees hurt when I do squats. What can I do?

First of all before beginning any kind of exercise program you should always see your doctor first to ensure that you are in good health. Having said that focus on modifying your technique. One issue may be that you are leaning too far forward on the downward motion. Try straightening your back as much as possible. Try keeping your heels on the ground when you squat can also help. You may also want to try performing a static exercise like the wall chair in order to build up your tendons and ligaments first.

I really want a 6-pack. If I put extra effort into core exercises can I get one?

Performing core exercises will make your abdominals stronger but they will not give you a 6-pack by themselves. In order to expose your abdominal muscles you have to lose fat and that means eating a clean diet. It simply isn't possible to perform an exercise in order to engage in spot reduction. It's not possible to lose fat in a specific area by exercising that one area. You may tone it so that it looks tighter but you need to lose weight all over your body to get the results you want. Remember the old adage that you get stronger in the gym but leaner in the kitchen. If you want a 6-pack you need to watch what you eat, no exceptions.

I have a hard time staying motivated. What can I do?

Follow your dream body blueprint. I know it may take a leap of faith but trust me on this; I didn't include that section no goal setting for no reason. In order to stay motivated you need to stay focused on your goals. You need to keep your subconscious and conscious minds working together by constantly thinking about and reading your goals everyday. Think about your dream body picture while you're doing your workouts. If you stick with this plan you will succeed.

Further Reading – Books On The Law Of Attraction

Think and Grow Rich by Napoleon Hill

The Science of Getting Rich by Wallace Wattles

The Law of Psychic Phenomena by Thomson Jay Hudson

The Laws of Manifestation by David Spangler

The Dynamic Laws of Prosperity by Catherine Ponder

Spiritual Economics by Eric Butterworth

Prosperity by Charles Fillmore

The Game of Life and How to Play It by Florence Scovel Shinn

Eight Pillars of Prosperity by James Allen

The Master Key System by Charles T. Hannel

The Success System that Never Fails by William Clement Stone

It Works by RHJ

Use the Power of Your Subconscious Mind To Obtain the Prosperity You Desire by Joseph Murphy

About The Author

Anthony Anholt has been interested and involved in athletics and fitness for his entire life. His specialty is "gym less" workouts, or exercise systems that do not require any kind of special equipment. He is also interested in enhancing performance in all sports, but particularly basketball. This is his second book.

About The Models

Bry Jensen is a Vancouver based fitness model, personal trainer and author. Bry is available for fitness, glamour and commercial modeling work. She can be reached through her website at bryjensen.com or on Facebook at facebook.com/Bry.Jensen.Fitness

Jordan Rayburn is a Vancouver based fitness competitor and model. He can be reached through his Facebook page at facebook.com/jordan.rayburn

One Last Thing

You've now reached the end of the book and I hope you find it useful in building a better you. If you did find it useful I would very much appreciate it if you could take 5 minutes and write a short review for it on Amazon or wherever you purchased it. Even a couple of sentences would be immensely helpful to me. Regardless I want to thank-you once again for purchasing my book and I wish you all the best in the future.

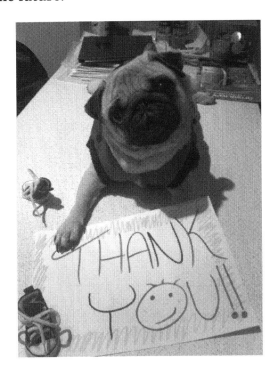